NO ORDINARY

JUICE

BOOK

NATASHA MAE SAYLISS OF
MAE + HARVEY

PAVILION

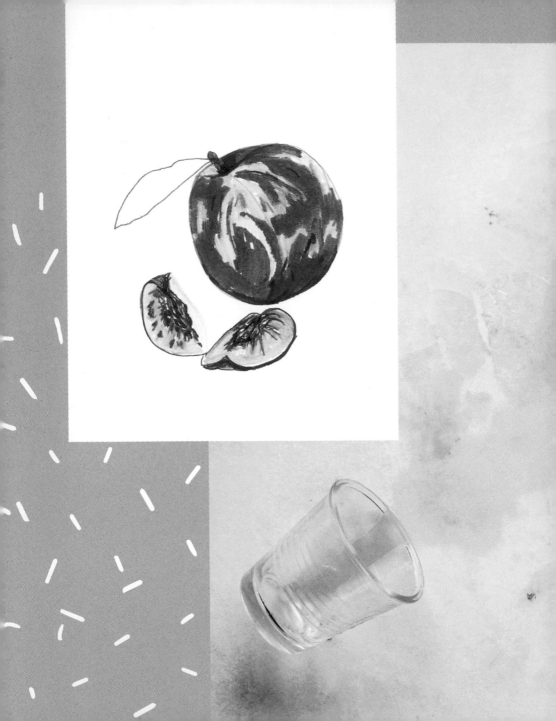

CONTENTS

INTRODUCTION

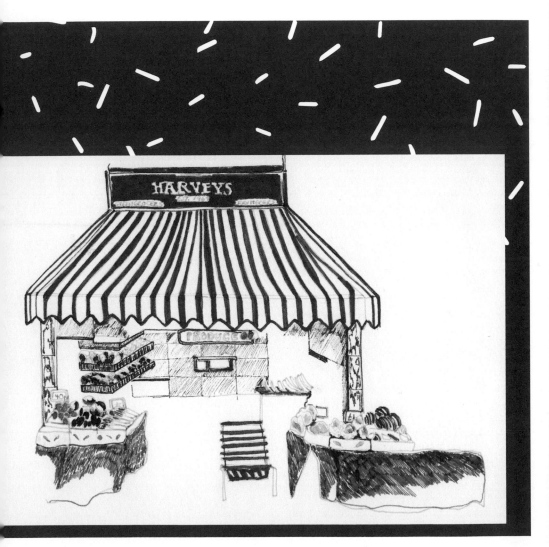

I decided to start making juices because there was nothing available to buy that was as fresh as the home-made my Grandma makes. I love knowing that the juices I sell are simple and that anybody can make them. They are just fruit and vegetables juiced, they haven't been pasteurised to extend their shelf life, so all the health benefits are intact; they haven't been diluted and nothing is added. When you take the time to make your own drinks, you know exactly what you've put into them.

Sadly, juicing these days is too often pushed into the 'health' sector. But we shouldn't be juicing out of a sense of duty; juices should be made for pleasure, to create something delicious. (I do have a juice recipe in this book containing kale, but just the one, and there are lots of cocktails and hot boozy drinks, too…)

I hope I've created juice recipes that you wouldn't have thought of yourself, and that actually taste fabulous rather than resembling a swamp! And the great thing about the recipes in this book are that they are just guidelines; they won't go too wrong unless you add ingredients that don't complement each other.

I've always tried to make my recipes as friendly as possible, so anybody of any age can enjoy them. I use what is in season, and I hope this book encourages you to shop at your local greengrocer rather than in the big supermarkets that stock everything all year round… it's more exciting this way, better for the environment AND cheaper.

But first, let me tell you how I got into juicing…

ABOUT MAE + HARVEY

My Grandpa Eric built all his granddaughters a dolls' house for our fifth birthdays. My sister and cousins received traditional dolls' houses, but I was given a baby blue-painted shop with 'Natasha Mae Sayliss Greengrocers, Established 1991' written on the shop sign. I guess the days of playing pretend shopkeeper with fruit and veg rubbed off on me.

I grew up in Wanstead, East London. Wanstead has a great high street, luckily still home to a greengrocer, fishmonger and other independent shops. Growing up, I always dreamed of having an all-day café there serving hearty food, then cocktails in the evenings and at weekends. With hindsight, I probably should have gone to cookery school, or studied something business-related, but that's not how it worked out.

Instead I took a Fashion Retail diploma. We were sent out on work placements, which were rather dull, but I always liked the customer service side: talking to people… and I still do. I then took a Painting degree and, at the same time, worked at the famous Borough Market for Boston Sausage and for Bear's Rotisserie, which I loved. The market influenced my paintings; they became more colourful and brighter. One of the best things about painting is going to an art shop and picking out paint colours; I get the same feeling when I shop for food, it's the excitement of sourcing items to create something that is going to be vibrant, colourful and tasty.

After graduating, I got an office job. On my way to work one morning, I got a text from my Grandma asking what I wanted for my birthday. As a child, one of the most exciting things about staying at Grandma's was the freshly squeezed orange juice in the morning. Still is! So I asked her for a juicer. I didn't get one; I got a smoothie maker instead (same thing, isn't it?!). However, when it arrived, inspiration came with it.

I came up with the idea of making fresh juices and smoothies to sell. I knew I needed to pick up more skills before jumping right in, so I decided to go back to Borough Market. That's when I started to work at Scotchtails, a scotch egg stall founded by Dom and Ollie, who have become a big part of Mae + Harvey. Looking around, I saw that the greengrocers at the market sold bottled juices, advertised as 'fresh'… but how could they be truly fresh with a long shelf life? I'd noticed a gap in the market.

So I went to see Peter, owner of JD Harvey, the greengrocer on Wanstead High Street, where he has worked since he was 15. (He's old now. Sorry, Pete!) Ever since I was little, my Dad and I would go shopping there on a Saturday for our fruit and veg, and we still do. So when I asked Peter if he could get me some ingredients from New Spitalfield's wholesale fruit and veg market - and if I could sell juices at his shop - he happily agreed. I wanted to collaborate with him and I wanted to name the drinks 'Mae + Harvey'. He probably thought I was bonkers…

We started in June 2014. In the beginning I just wanted to see if people were interested in buying my drinks. I ordered glass bottles and label stickers. My friend Kenny designed the labels; he also came up with the logo, which I loved from the start. I selected the flavours, borrowed my neighbour's juicer and put my smoothie machine from Grandma into service.

On that first Saturday, Mum and I were up at the crack of dawn, making juices and smoothies, then bottling and labelling each one. I got to the shop two hours later than planned. Pete had set up a little pitch for me, and I stood there encouraging people to try the drinks, while my older sister Alex stood outside saying 'Mmmm… this is delicious!' In fact my sister has come to every market since and bought a juice. She is my biggest fan… so thank you, Alex!

At first, the bottles looked really vibrant, but slowly the labels turned brown, and began to peel off. Nevertheless, I had sold a few and people seemed intrigued, so that made me even more excited about giving Mae + Harvey a proper go. It wasn't until after that first day that I started to research juicing, the difference between juices and smoothies, and cold-pressed versus fresh (I did it the wrong way round).

After selling juices at Harvey's every Saturday that summer, I became a bit more confident. I bought a household cold-press juicer, which made such a difference to the juices; I even got them stocked in a couple of pubs on the high street. I sold them from market stalls, first at the new Village Green Market in Hackney Downs, then at Netil Market in London Fields. I loved it! It was great being around successful traders. But it made me realise that I also wanted to sell soups, pickles and other things made from fresh produce, so I decided to go down the wholesale route.

For the first year, I was making juices in my parents' kitchen, turning their tile grouting shades of purple, green and orange – much to their delight – and driving around London dropping off samples to retailers. I started to get some stockists but they didn't take many juices, mostly because they were expensive and had a short shelf life, two things that standard retailers dislike. Plus, it took me ages to make the juices, as I was still using two small domestic juicers. So when Dom and Ollie from Scotchtails decided to open a coffee shop, Lundenwic, a stone's throw from Covent Garden, they helped me buy a commercial juicer and allowed me to make the drinks in the kitchen there, which made everything so much easier; suddenly, it felt like a 'proper' business.

There have been lots of changes with my juices – the look, where they are made, where the fruit and veg are sourced and where they are sold – but what hasn't changed is the recipes and how they are made. It's just fruit and veg, juiced.

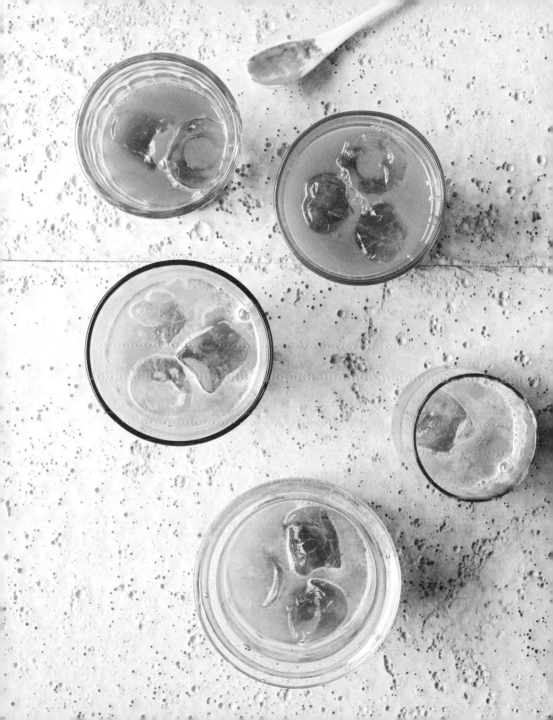

HARDWARE

Before you start, it is important to have the right machine
for you. Juicers aren't cheap and you want to be using
them often; you don't want an appliance that just sits in
your cupboard, gathering dust. So which should you buy?

CITRUS JUICER
Essential. You'll be able to make a lot of the recipes in this
book just with one of these.

CENTRIFUGAL JUICER
Quick to use and easy to clean. However, they aren't
great at juicing leafy greens, berries or herbs, as too
much heat is generated from the fast-rotating blades and
fruits and vegetables get damaged quickly. The outcome is a
juice with too much foam, that needs to be sieved straight
away to achieve a smoother, less foamy drink. The juices
last 48 hours, but they need shaking, and they do turn
brown. Nevertheless, if drunk straight away, your body
can enjoy the nutrients that remain.

MASTICATING JUICER

Also known as a 'slow juicer', this chews up fruits
and vegetables slowly, so the juice is richer in nutrients
and flavour. I started Mae + Harvey using one of these.
I found the juice I made with it had a shelf life of up to
three days and the colours were vibrant because there isn't
as much heat involved in the process. (It's heat that damages
nutrients.) Most of these juicers are more expensive, the
juice takes longer to make and the machine to clean up.
But quite a lot of my recipes can be doubled and have that
three-day shelf life, so really you only have to get your
juicer out once or twice a week.

COLD-PRESS JUICER

These have two separate components: a grinder and a press.
The first grinds the ingredients into a pulp that is then
transferred into cloths. These are pressed against two metal
plates under enormous pressure, which creates no heat; the
result is a juice with a huge amount of nutrients (25 times
more than with any other juicer) and flavour. The colour and
taste is amazing and you get 50 per cent more juice from the
ingredients than with any other type of juicer. I hope this
helps you understand why cold-pressed juices are expensive.
When I first started using one, I was still running the
business from home; you can still see the remains of an
exploding cloth full of beetroot pulp on my parents' kitchen
tiles... Very, very messy!

JUICING TIPS AND INGREDIENTS

STAIN PREVENTION
Always make sure you wear an **apron** and cover your surfaces before you start juicing. Take your crisp white shirt off anyway before you begin!

STEADY THE MACHINE
Place a couple of **tea towels** underneath your juicer; this will obviously make clean-up slightly easier and keep your machine steady.

CLEAN THE PRODUCE
Fill a sink with cold water and a good squeeze of lemon juice, then drop your ingredients into it and give them a good clean.

PREPARE THE INGREDIENTS
Chop the ingredients to whatever size they need to be to fit down your juicer chute.

IF YOU'RE USING LEAFY GREENS…
…it is always good to put in a cucumber, or something else with a high water content, straight after the leaves, to help push them down. Usually everything else seems to be fine, chuck it down the juicer chute in whatever order you fancy.

TASTE IT!
Once you have made a juice, have a **taste** and – if you want to add an extra bit of something – go for it (and remember that lemon or lime juice and even sea salt help to bring out the other flavours). Sieve the juice into another jug to remove bits if you like, pour into your glass and enjoy!

KEEPING JUICES
If you have scaled up a recipe and made larger quantities because you want to **keep** the juice for a bit longer, seal

it into glass airtight containers. They should stay fresh in the fridge for up to 4 days if you have made them in a masticating ('slow') juicer, or 48 hours if they were made using a centrifugal machine. (Though I find green juices have the best flavour straight after making.)

GLUTS
When making juices, it's cheapest to buy seasonal produce and, as this can often be a bargain, I find I often have a few things left over, or buy more than I need. So I have included a few non-juice recipes in each season: either favourite recipes that my friends and family make, or a few that I like making myself. These are all fruit- and vegetable-based but can complement different foods and occasions. My Dad's side of the family are Jewish and my Grandma has given me a few of her greatest pickling recipes, which are fantastic for using up gluts.

BUY THE BEST YOU CAN
I have grown up surrounded by people who love food, thinking about what I am going to eat today – and what my next meal is going to be – and if I have a bad meal, it ruins my day! I think knowing what is in your food and drink is really important, even if it is a cheeky cake or a soda with sugar, at least when it's home-made you know how much you're having and what's in it.

WHERE TO SHOP
It is great to shop around for your produce. I like to go to Chinese and international supermarkets, it's where I buy things that are slightly tropical: they are cheaper and the quality is just as good. They sell ingredients such as pomelos, papayas, coconuts, hibiscus and rose petals, huge watermelons, Asian pears and pineapples. Other than that, there's very little in this book that your local greengrocer won't have! So let's get going…

SPRING

It's always great when spring comes along, the days get longer and we come out of hibernation! Spring is also a reminder that summer is on its way. For this season I have included some refreshing juices, a great chilled soup, some salads and a number of shrubs (and no, they aren't little bushes)… keep reading and you will soon find out.

PAPAYAS

JUICE
PAPAYA + LIME

A winning combination of
sweet and sour. If you're
having trouble finding papayas
in your local supermarket,
try and find an international
store, as they are normally
in plentiful supply there.

Serves 1

1 papaya
1 lime, zest and pith removed
   (reserve a slice for
   garnish if you wish)

JUICE
GREEN PAPAYA,
CUCUMBER + APPLE

Serves 1

1 green papaya, peeled and
   seeds removed
1 medium-sized cucumber,
   unpeeled
1 green apple, unpeeled
1 tsp raw agave syrup
1 tsp ground cinnamon
a handful of mint

1 Juice the papaya first,
   along with the cucumber
   and apple.

2 Mix in the agave syrup and
   ground cinnamon.

3 Add the mint to the glass
   and pour the juice over
   to serve.

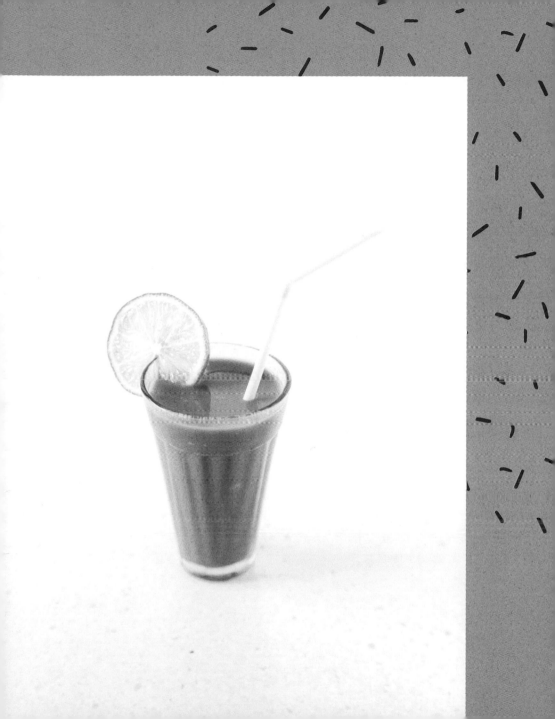

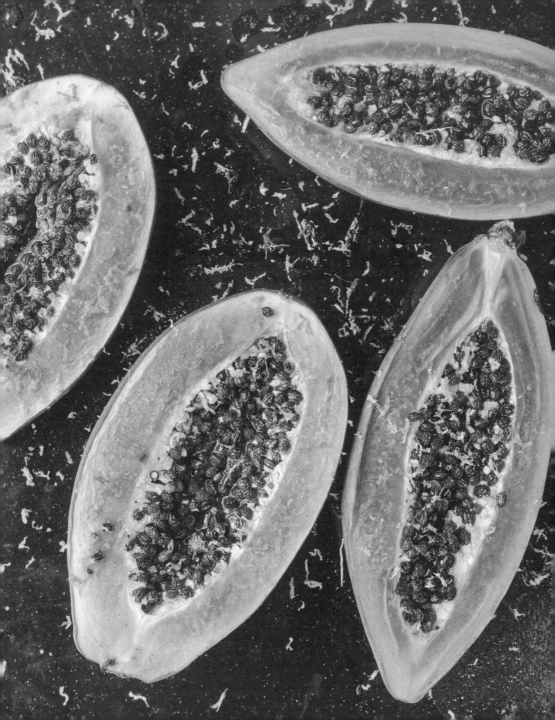

RECIPE
ROASTED PAPAYA WITH HONEY + LIME

A refreshing dessert, treat yourself and serve it with
a scoop of vanilla ice cream.

Serves 4 as a small treat

2 papayas, halved and deseeded
4 tsp honey, or to taste
juice of 1 lime, or to taste

1 Preheat the oven to 180°C/350°F/gas 4.

2 Place each papaya half in a baking dish, drizzle 1 tsp of
  honey on each half and generously squeeze the lime over.
  Bake until soft enough that the flesh can be easily scooped
  out of the skin; depending on the size of the papaya, this
  could take 20-45 minutes. Baste the papayas in the juices
  every so often.

3 Add more honey and lime to taste, then serve.

SHRUBS

The word "shrub" is derived from the Arabic *sharbah*, which means "a drink". "Sherbet" and "syrup" also come from this Arabic root.

When I started this book, I wanted to try and recreate old-fashioned drinks, and this section provides the perfect example. Also known as drinking vinegar, a shrub is a syrup, like a cordial, and making a shrub at home is a great way of preserving and experimenting with seasonal fruit. You could also use the syrups in salad dressings, home-made jams (jellies), or as a glaze.

My Nan used to make shrubs, and we managed to find her old recipes! Me and my friend Florence have created some cool flavours for you to try.

For a shrub to be successful, you need to use fruits that are ripe and sweet. You can use any vinegar as long as it has at least 5 per cent acidity. Before you start you need:

A sterilised 1 litre/1 quart glass jar (see page 159)
A saucepan
Cheesecloth (or use a nut milk bag/straining bag)

All of these are shrubs made in exactly the same way, with the fruit (and flavourings, such as ginger and pink peppercorns), added to the sterilised jar first. For all of these recipes, you will need to start 4 weeks in advance.

All make 700ml/1½ pints/3 cups

For method, see pages 24-25.

RASPBERRY + APPLE CIDER VINEGAR SHRUB

250g/9oz raspberries
480ml/17fl oz/2 cups apple cider vinegar
250g/9oz/1¼ cups brown sugar

NECTARINE, GINGER + CHAMPAGNE VINEGAR SHRUB

250g/9oz nectarines, halved, pitted and chopped
15g/0.4oz/¼ cup root ginger, peeled and finely grated
480ml/17fl oz/2 cups Champagne vinegar
250g/9oz/1¼ cups brown sugar

ASIAN PEAR, PINK PEPPERCORN + WHITE WINE VINEGAR SHRUB

250g/9oz Asian pears, cored and chopped
1 tsp pink peppercorns
480ml/17fl oz/2 cups white wine vinegar
250g/9oz/1¼ cups brown sugar

STRAWBERRY + BALSAMIC VINEGAR SHRUB

250g/9oz strawberries, hulled
480ml/17fl oz/2 cups balsamic vinegar
250g/9oz/1¼ cups brown sugar

1 Place the fruit (and ginger or peppercorns, where necessary) into a sterilised jar (see page 159).

2 Heat the vinegar in a saucepan, but don't let it boil. Pour the vinegar over the fruit, leaving a small gap at the top of the jar. Make sure the rim of the jar is clean and seal the lid on tightly.

3 Let the vinegar cool completely, then store the jar in your fridge, while the flavours infuse.

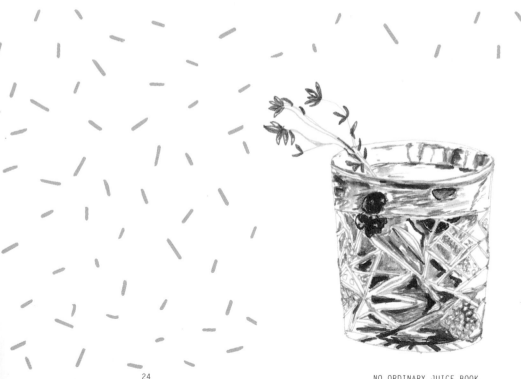

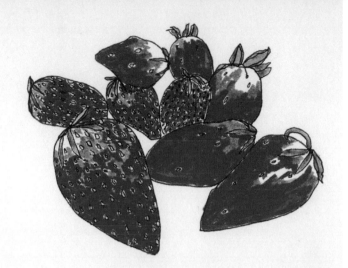

...4 weeks later

1 Strain the fruit from the vinegar through damp cheesecloth, or a nut milk bag. Repeat if necessary, to remove any last pieces of fruit or flavourings. The leftover fruit is now great for chutneys... or the bin!

5 Place the infused vinegar and the sugar into a saucepan. Bring to the boil, stirring so the sugar dissolves. Once dissolved, remove from the heat and let it cool. Pour into a clean, sterilised jar (see page 159) and seal the lid on tightly.

6 Store the shrub in the fridge, and it should last up to 6 months.

7 When you are finally ready to serve, mix 1 tbsp of shrub syrup into a glass of still or sparkling water and taste, adding more syrup if desired. You could also add the raspberry shrub to a gin and tonic, while the nectarine and Asian pear versions are nice with a glass of fizz.

LASSIS

Lassis are yogurt-based drinks from India, traditionally made from yogurt, water, spices and sometimes fruit. The most basic version is a savoury drink flavoured with ground roasted cumin. I have created sweeter lassis… which means lassis with fruits!

SWEET LASSI WITH ROSE WATER

Serves 2

½ tsp rose water
360ml/12fl oz/1½ cups natural yogurt
3 tbsp brown sugar
1 tsp edible dried rose petals

1 Place all the ingredients except the rose petals in a blender with 120ml/4fl oz/½ cup of ice-cold water. Blend until smooth.

2 Serve over ice, sprinkling the dried rose petals on top.

PEACH + PISTACHIO LASSI

Serves 2

2 peaches, halved and pitted
2 tbsp shelled, unsalted pistachios
120ml/4fl oz/½ cup Greek yogurt
1 tsp ground cinnamon
1 tbsp honey

Blend all the ingredients together with 120ml/4fl oz/½ cup of ice-cold water and serve over ice.

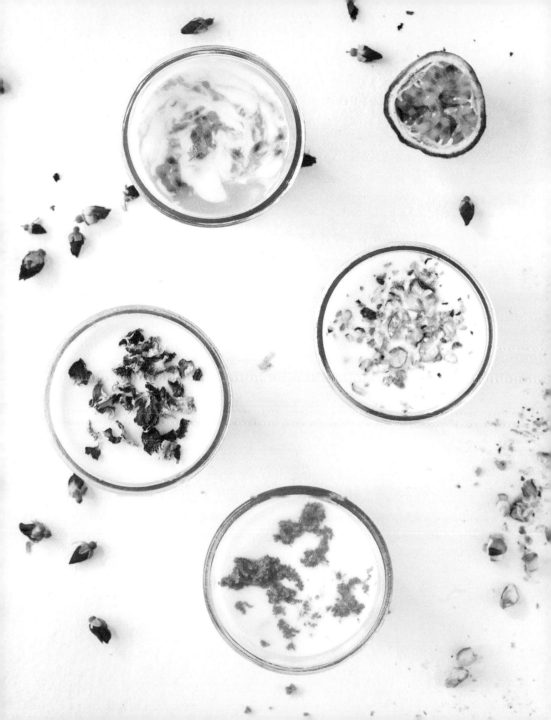

CANTALOUPE + LIME LASSI

Serves 2

½ cantaloupe, seeds
  and skin removed
120ml/4fl oz/½ cup natural
  yogurt
1 tsp cayenne pepper
juice of 1 lime

1 Blend everything apart
  from the lime juice with
  120ml/4fl oz/½ cup of
  ice-cold water.

2 Once the ingredients in the
  blender are smooth, squeeze
  in the lime juice and serve
  over ice.

MANGO, PAPAYA + COCONUT LASSI

**If you shut your eyes while
you're drinking this lassi,
the tropical flavours will
make you feel as if you're on
a beach somewhere far away!**

Serves 2 (drink immediately)

½ mango, peeled, pitted
  and chopped
1 papaya, skinned, deseeded
  and chopped
120ml/4fl oz/½ cup coconut
  yogurt

Blend all the ingredients
together with 120ml/4fl oz/
½ cup of ice-cold water and
serve over ice.

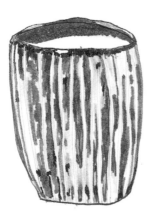

RHUBARB + ORANGE LASSI

We have two seasons for rhubarb in the UK; December to March gives us forced rhubarb (it's grown in the dark in sheds). The other is from April to September and this is when we get the main crop of outdoor-grown rhubarb. An interesting fact for you: rhubarb isn't actually a fruit. It's a vegetable! Who knew?!

Serves 2

200g/7oz rhubarb
finely grated zest and juice
   of 1 orange
4 tbsp honey
1 tsp orange blossom water
120ml/4fl oz/½ cup natural
   yogurt

1 Cook the rhubarb over a low heat with the orange zest and juice and the honey; simmer until the rhubarb is soft. Once soft, tip the rhubarb into a sieve placed over a bowl. (Keep the juices as, once cool, they become a lovely cordial that you can have with ice and water.)

2 Once the rhubarb is completely cool, blend it with the rest of the ingredients and 120ml/ 4fl oz/½ cup of ice-cold water. Serve over ice.

SCENTED MELONS

JUICE
HONEYDEW MELON, RHUBARB
+ ORANGE

The melon juice is hydrating
and soothing, the rhubarb
brings tartness and the
orange just makes it easy to
drink again.

Serves 2

½ melon, seeds and
   skin removed
200g/7oz rhubarb
1 orange, zest and
   pith removed

JUICE
CANTALOUPE, ORANGE + TURMERIC

Both cantaloupe and oranges
are loaded with vitamin C, so
this is a great drink to give
you a bit of a boost. The
turmeric brings all the warm
flavours together and creates
a lovely bright drink.

Serves 2

½ cantaloupe, seeds and
   skin removed
1 orange, zest and
   pith removed
1 tsp ground turmeric

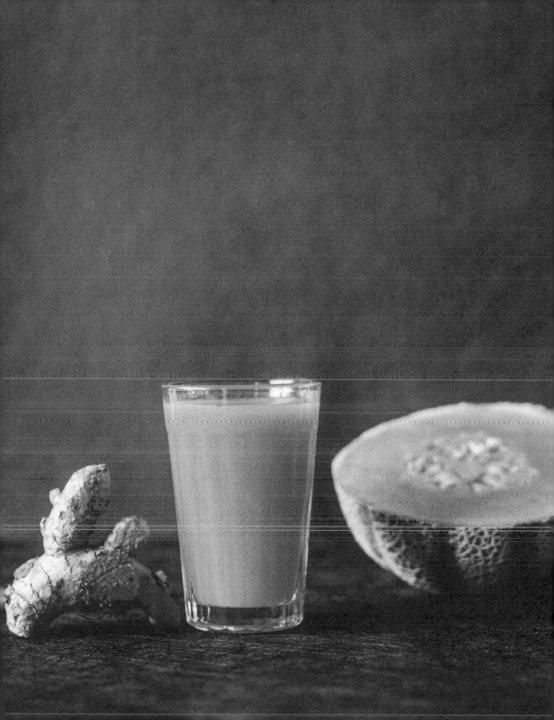

RECIPE
CANTALOUPE CHILLED SOUP

Although chilled soups are popular, it isn't often you see
a chilled sweet soup. This could be served as a starter,
as a palate cleanser between courses, or for dessert with
yogurt or ice cream.

Serves 2

1 orange, zest and pith removed
1 nectarine, pitted
¼ lime, zest and pith removed
½ cantaloupe, seeds and skin removed
½ tbsp maple syrup
¼ tsp ground cinnamon
¼ tsp sea salt
4 leaves of mint

1 First make a blend of citrus juice. Juice the orange,
  nectarine and lime together. You should have about 250ml/
  9fl oz/1 cup of juice.

2 Place it in a blender with all the other ingredients.
  Blend until smooth.

RECILE

RECIPE
CANTALOUPE, CUCUMBER, RADISH + BASIL SALAD

This is a very fresh, light and beautiful spring salad, which is also really easy to make.

Serves 4 as a starter

½ cantaloupe, seeds and skin removed, cut into small chunks
1 cucumber, halved lengthways, deseeded and sliced
4 radishes, sliced very thinly, ideally on a mandolin
8 big basil leaves, rolled together and shredded
1 tbsp extra virgin olive oil
½ tbsp balsamic vinegar
sea salt and freshly ground black pepper

1 Toss all the ingredients together into a bowl.

2 Season with sea salt and freshly ground black pepper.

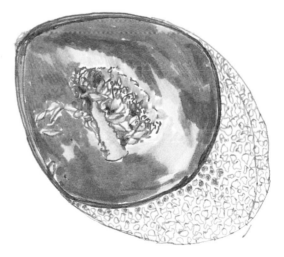

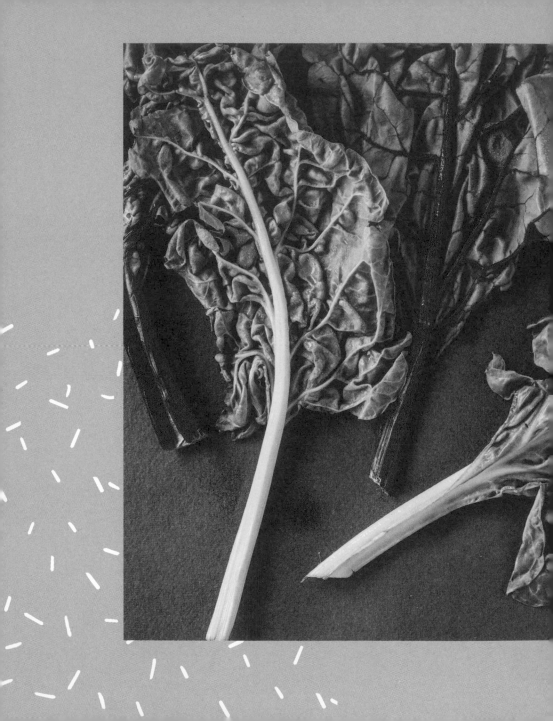

JUICE
RAINBOW CHARD, HONEYDEW
MELON, FENNEL, COURGETTE
+ LEMON

One of those juices which
you might find intimidating,
but don't knock it till you
try it; chard is highly
nutritious and melon is
super-hydrating!

Serves 2

¼ honeydew melon
½ fennel bulb
1 courgette (zucchini)
1 lemon, zest and
  pith removed
100g/3½oz rainbow chard

JUICE
HONEYDEW MELON + PEAR

A mellow and sweet juice.

Serves 2

½ honeydew melon, seeds and
  skin removed
2 pears

PINEAPPLES

JUICE
BEETROOT, PINEAPPLE + GINGER

Pineapples remind me of summer, but they are available in springtime, too; they are slightly more expensive but they are super-sweet. This juice combination is a popular one; it always goes down well in the spring as you still get the warming qualities from the ginger and the thickness from the beetroot. The pineapple nicely sweetens it. Beetroots (beets) hold all sorts of nutrients, and are thought to be able to reduce blood pressure.

Serves 2

3 raw beetroots (beets), peeled and chopped
¼ pineapple, peeled and chopped
thumb-sized chunk of root ginger, peeled

RECIPE
ROASTED PINEAPPLE WITH LIME + VANILLA

I have a serious sweet tooth - a lot of people do -
so I often crave something sweet after a meal. This
shouldn't make you feel too guilty afterwards, either.

Serves 6

1 pineapple, topped and tailed, hard skin sliced off
finely grated zest of 1 lime, plus the juice of 2
4 tbsp maple syrup
seeds from 1 vanilla pod

1 Preheat the oven to 200°C/400°F/gas 6.

2 Slice the pineapple into 2cm/½in thick rounds and lay
  them on a baking dish.

3 In a small bowl, mix together the lime zest and
  juice, the maple syrup and vanilla seeds, then pour
  over the pineapple.

4 Roast for around 45 minutes, basting every so often.

5 Eat hot.

POMELOS

JUICE
POMELO

Pomelos are the largest fruit in the citrus family, primarily found in South-East Asia. I came across them in a Chinese supermarket; apparently they are great for digestion and the immune system, too. So this super-tasty juice is delicious and healthy!

Serves 2

1 pomelo, zest and pith removed

DRINK
POMELO, JALAPEÑO + TEQUILA COCKTAIL

If you can't get hold of pomelos, this cocktail is just as good with pink grapefruit. If you don't like things hot, this might not be the one for you! Todd, I have made this for you… I know how much you love tequila and jalapeños.

Serves 2

For the jalapeño-infused syrup
2 jalapeños, halved
finely grated zest of 1 pomelo
200g/7oz/1 cup granulated sugar

For the cocktail
400ml/14fl oz/1¾ cups pomelo juice
100ml/3½fl oz/scant ½ cup lime juice
2 shots of tequila

1 Start by making the syrup: in a saucepan, combine the jalapeño, pomelo zest, sugar and 240ml/8fl oz/1 cup of water. Bring to a simmer, stirring to dissolve the sugar.

2 Once the sugar has dissolved, remove from the heat, strain into a bowl and cool. Once cool, store in a sterilised jar (see page 159). This will keep for 1 week if you want to make it in advance.

3 To make the cocktail, combine 15ml/1 tbsp of the infused syrup with all the other ingredients in a cocktail shaker and shake with ice. Serve over ice.

RHUBARB

DRINK
RHUBARB LEMONADE SODA

One of my favourite rhubarb drinks and a great one to make
when you have a few friends round on a nice sunny spring
day (when we have them). This also makes a great mixer for
a refreshing gin cocktail.

Serves 6

750g/1lb 10oz rhubarb, chopped
150g/5½oz/¾ cup granulated sugar
long strips of lemon zest
4 sprigs of mint, plus more to serve
240ml/8fl oz/1 cup freshly squeezed lemon juice
sparkling water, to serve

1 In a saucepan, stir together the rhubarb, sugar, lemon zest
  and mint with 1 litre/1¾ pints of cold water. Bring to the
  boil, stirring until the sugar dissolves. Reduce the heat,
  cover and simmer for 15 minutes.

2 Let the rhubarb mixture cool, strain it through a sieve over
  a large jug and press on the mixture to extract as much
  liquid as possible. Top the liquid up with the lemon juice
  and sparkling water.

3 Serve over ice with a fresh sprig of mint. Add an optional
  shot of gin if desired!

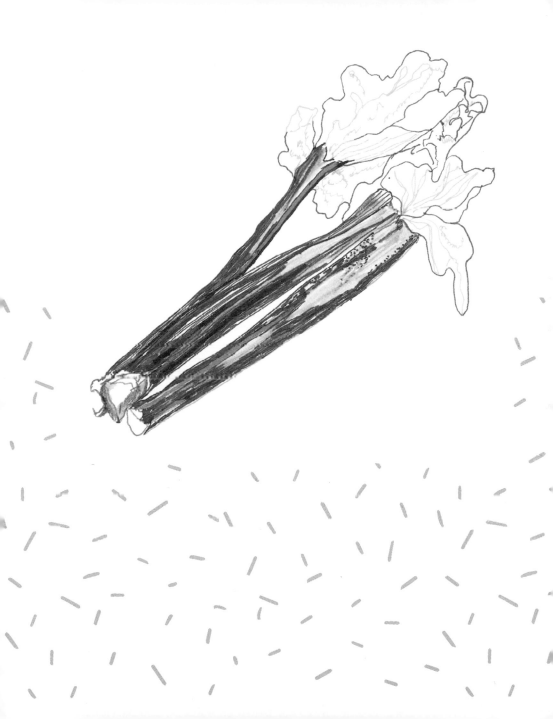

RECIPE
NAOMI'S RHUBARB + ORANGE CAKE

My boyfriend George has a wonderful Grandma and she is also
very good at baking. I wanted a rhubarb cake and she happened
to have a recipe up her sleeve!

Serves 8-10

For the cake
350g/12oz rhubarb, cut into 3.5cm/1½in lengths
225g/8oz/generous 1 cup golden caster (superfine) sugar
finely grated zest and juice of ½ small orange
140g/5oz/⅔ cup unsalted butter, softened, plus
  more for the tin
2 eggs, lightly beaten
½ tsp baking powder
85g/3oz/⅔ cup self-raising (self-rising) flour
115g/4oz/1¼ cup ground almonds

For the topping
30g/1oz/2 tbsp unsalted butter
30g/1oz/scant 2½ tbsp light muscovado sugar
finely grated zest of ½ small orange
55g/2oz/½ cup flaked (slivered) almonds

1 Mix the rhubarb with 55g/2oz/¼ cup of the caster (superfine)
  sugar and the orange zest. Set aside for 1 hour, stirring
  once or twice.

2 Preheat the oven to 190°C/375°F/gas 5. Butter a 23cm/9in
  diameter, 7.5cm/3in deep loose-bottomed cake tin and line
  the base with baking parchment.

3 Cream the butter and remaining caster (superfine) sugar in
  a bowl until fluffy. Add the eggs, baking powder, flour and
  ground almonds. Beat gently until smooth, taking care not

to over-mix. Stir in the orange juice, spoon into the tin and level with a spoon. Drain the rhubarb in a sieve over a bowl. Spoon the chunks over the base. Bake for 25 minutes.

4 Reduce the oven to 180°C/350°F/gas 4. For the topping, melt the butter, then stir in the sugar, zest and almonds. Sprinkle over the cake and cook for 20 minutes, or until firm in the centre. Cool in the tin for 20 minutes, then transfer to a wire rack and peel off the baking parchment.

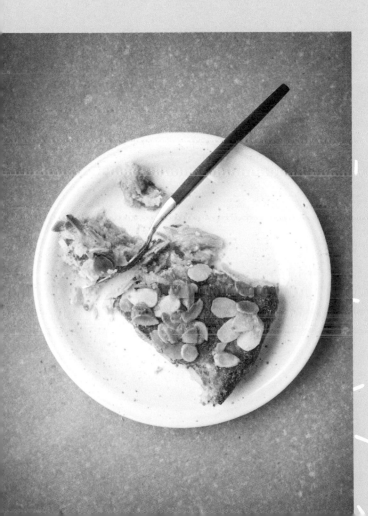

RECIPE
ROASTED RHUBARB + STRAWBERRY COMPOTE WITH VANILLA + CINNAMON FRENCH TOAST

The best brunch known to (wo)man. To make it extra special, serve with extra-crispy bacon.

Serves 4

For the compote
150g/5½oz strawberries
150g/5½oz rhubarb
1 tbsp balsamic vinegar
4 tbsp maple syrup
1 tsp sea salt

For the toast
4 eggs
600ml/21fl oz/generous 2½ cups milk
sea salt
2 tsp ground cinnamon
seeds from 2 vanilla pods
30g/1oz/2 tbsp unsalted butter, softened
6 slices of challah bread/white tin loaf, thickly sliced

1 For the compote, preheat the oven to 180°C/350°F/gas 4. Line a baking tray with baking parchment.

2 In a large bowl, mix the strawberries and rhubarb. In a separate small bowl, whisk together the balsamic vinegar, maple syrup and salt. Pour this over the rhubarb and strawberries and mix together. Spread the fruit out on the baking tray in a single layer and drizzle the remaining juices all over the fruit.

3 Roast for 30 minutes. The juices should be thick and the fruit should be tender. Transfer to a bowl once out of the oven and still warm.

4 On to the toast. In a large bowl, whisk together the eggs, milk, salt, ground cinnamon and half the vanilla. Transfer to a shallow dish.

5 Scrape the remaining vanilla seeds into the butter and, with clean hands or a fork, mix them together.

6 Dip both sides of the bread into the egg mixture.

7 Melt 1 tbsp of the vanilla butter in a non-stick frying pan over a medium-high heat. Fry the slices of bread until golden on one side, then turn and fry the other side. Keep the French toast warm while you fry the rest of the bread, adding more butter if you need it.

SPRING CITRUS

JUICE
PINK GRAPEFRUIT, ORANGE + TURMERIC

A Mae + Harvey spring classic! You can buy fresh turmeric
from international supermarkets and the colour and taste is
amazing. It is so soothing for your stomach and is thought to
help with arthritis and diabetes.

Serves 2

2 pink grapefruits, zest and pith removed
2 large oranges, zest and pith removed
thumb-sized piece of turmeric, peeled

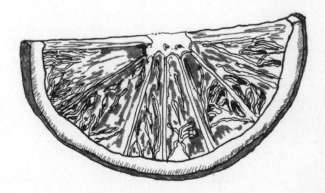

DRINK
GIN, PINK GRAPEFRUIT + ROSEMARY FIZZ COCKTAIL

This is a great twist on a classic gin and tonic, replacing the tonic water with Prosecco (or Champagne if you're feeling fancy!) and adding grapefruit juice. The rosemary adds great flavour and looks really pretty, too.

Serves 2

2 shots of gin
1 pink grapefruit, juiced
   (approx. 150ml/5fl oz/
   scant ⅔ cup)
fizz, to top up
2 sprigs of rosemary

1 Get a small glass jug and clink in a few ice cubes. Pour in the gin, followed by the pink grapefruit juice.

2 Top up with fizz and the rosemary and stir.

JUICE
BLUEBERRY, PEAR + LIME

We see blueberries used in smoothies more often than in juices, so here's a juice! The berries are great for the digestive and urinary systems!

Serves 2

2 pears
½ lime, zest and pith removed
150g/5½oz blueberries

SUMMER

The best season for cold and refreshing drinks. Last summer, I took part in Hackney Drinks Market, where I made cocktails from cold-pressed juices… they went down a treat! There's some here, so read on... I have also given you drinkable granitas, Italian iced creations traditionally made from sugar syrups. And keep your eyes peeled in this chapter for some lovely summery salads, sodas, pickles and puddings that are all great for summer barbecues.

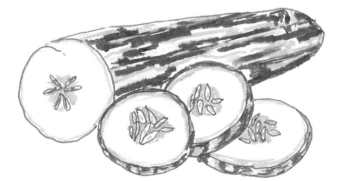

JUICE YOUR SALAD

JUICE
CELERY, KIWI, CORIANDER +
LIME (+ AVOCADO)

This juice reminds me of the
greatest dip ever to exist:
guacamole. Using the first
4 ingredients only, this
recipe can be a juice, but
you can also add the juice to
a blender with the avocado
to make a delicious and
filling smoothie.

Serves 1

4 celery sticks
4 kiwis, peeled
½ lime, zest and pith removed
20g/¾oz coriander
  (cilantro)
½ avocado (optional)

JUICE
CUCUMBER, GREEN GRAPE + BASIL

When I first started making
juices, I used a lot of
grapes as they are so
naturally sweet. However,
they are quite expensive,
so it is best to make
juices with grapes on a
smaller scale.

Serves 1

150g/5½oz cucumber
100g/3½oz green grapes
handful of basil

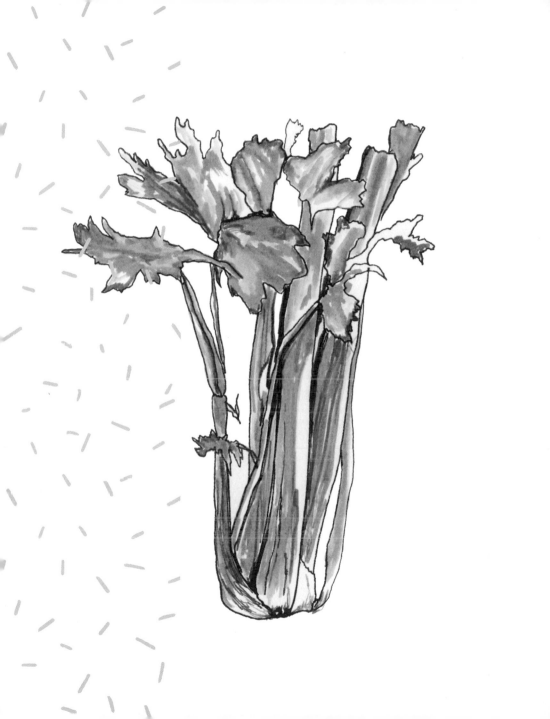

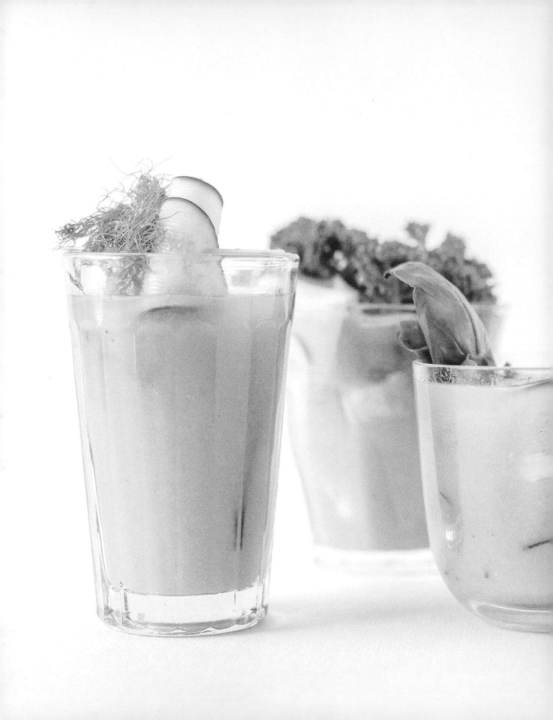

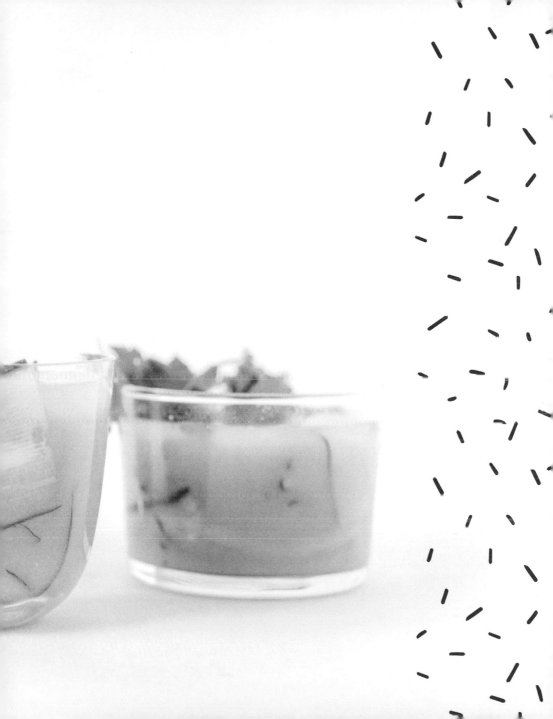

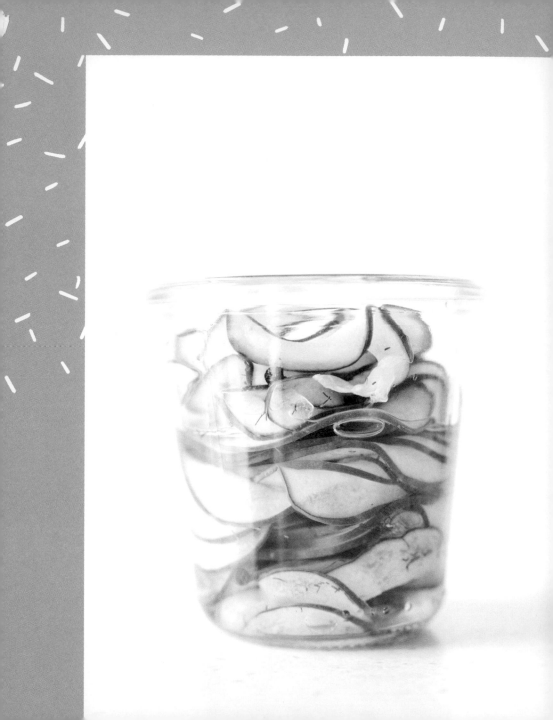

RECITE
PICKLED CUCUMBERS

Grandma Ruth's pickled cucumbers - a great addition to any salad, bagel or just on their own!

Makes 1 jar

1 medium cucumber
2 tsp sea salt
120ml/4fl oz/½ cup white wine vinegar
70g/2½oz/⅓ cup granulated sugar
2 tsp dill fronds
6 peppercorns
1 garlic clove
2 bay leaves

1 With a mandolin, slice the cucumber into thin rounds. Place it into a colander, sprinkle with the salt. Let the cucumbers strain in the salt for about 1 hour.

2 Get a glass bowl and pour in 120ml/4fl oz/½ cup of cold water. Add the vinegar and the sugar.

3 Rinse the salt off the cucumbers under running cold water, then submerge the slices in the pickle juice and mix in the dill, peppercorns, garlic cloves and bay leaves.

4 Place into a jar and put the lid on tightly. This will keep for 1 week.

PINEAPPLES

JUICE
PINEAPPLE + CHILLI

Teaming the pineapple with the red chilli, which is a very good source of vitamin C, this juice will help to reduce inflammation and build your immune system. For a less healthy option, you could also add a shot of rum!

Serves 2

1 pineapple, peeled and
  chopped
1 red chilli, halved
  and deseeded

DRINK
FROZEN PIÑA COLADA

The creamy real deal, garnished with fresh cherries and pineapple.

Serves 1

2 shots of dark rum
3 tbsp coconut cream
100ml/3½fl oz/scant ½ cup
  fresh pineapple juice
juice of ½ lime
1 cherry
1 pineapple wedge

1 Combine the rum, coconut cream, pineapple juice and lime juice in a blender. Add loads of ice cubes and blend until smooth.

2 Pour into glasses and add the cherry and the pineapple wedge.

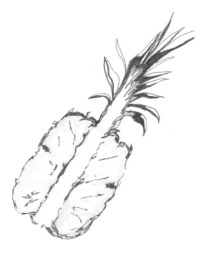

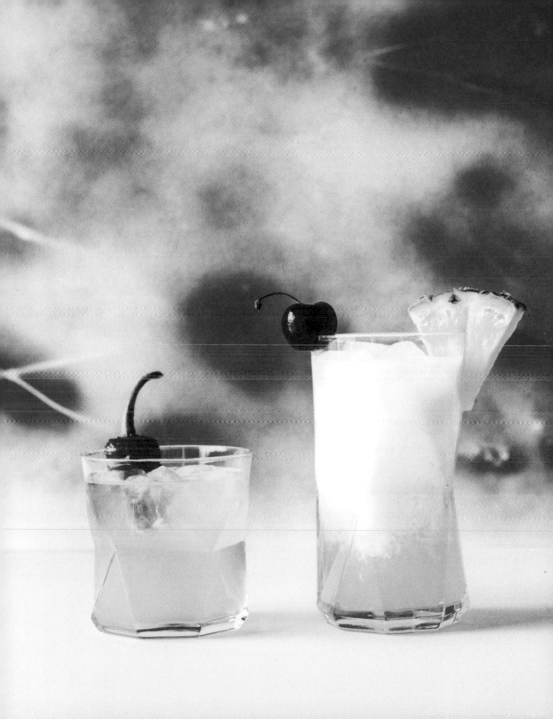

JUICE
PINEAPPLE + COCONUT

The flavours of this juice are influenced by the classic creamy
cocktail, the piña colada (see previous page). If you have
any international supermarkets nearby, they tend to have
young coconuts; however, you will need the right tools to get
the coconut open… alternatively, shop-bought coconut water
is pretty good these days!

Serves 2

1 pineapple, peeled and chopped
120ml/4fl oz/½ cup coconut water
80g/2¾oz fresh coconut pieces

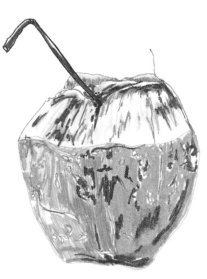

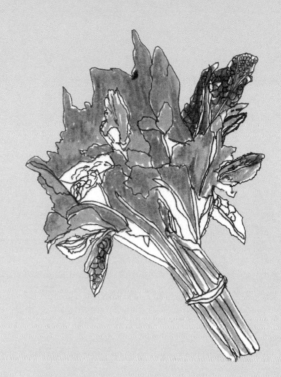

JUICE
PINEAPPLE, CUCUMBER, LIME + MINT

This juice is a Mae + Harvey summer special, the sweetest green juice in town! You could also add a shot of vodka.

Serves 2

1 pineapple, peeled and chopped
½ cucumber
¼ lime, zest and pith removed
6 mint leaves

INDIAN SUMMER

DRINK
GINGER BEER

My sister loves ginger beer. This isn't the traditional way of making it, but you get the best flavours from juicing the ginger with the lemon, which together hit the back of your throat (in a good way!). If it is a bit too sharp for your taste, add 1 teaspoon of honey to sweeten it. You could also add a shot of rum!

Serves 2

60g/2¼oz root ginger, peeled
1 lemon, zest and
   pith removed
200ml/7fl oz/scant 1 cup tonic
   water
4 mint leaves

1 Juice the ginger and
   the lemon.

2 Divide between 2 glasses,
   top up with the tonic water
   and serve over ice cubes
   with the mint leaves.

DRINK
TOMATO, MANGO + SUMAC LASSI

Mango is quite a popular ingredient in lassis; the tomato makes it savoury and the sumac brings a lemony taste (the spice is popular in Middle Eastern cooking).

Serves 2

240ml/8fl oz/1 cup Greek
   yogurt
75g/2½oz tomatoes, chopped
   (sweet and juicy ones)
75g/2½oz mango, cubed
½ tsp ground cardamom
½ tsp ground sumac,
   plus ½ tsp more to serve
½ tsp finely grated unwaxed
   lemon zest
1½ tbsp agave syrup
4 mint leaves

1 Combine all the ingredients
   except the mint leaves
   in a blender, adding
   3 ice cubes.

2 Serve with mint and a
   sprinkling more sumac.

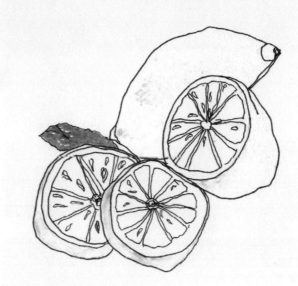

DRINK
PASSION FRUIT + AGAVE SYRUP LASSI

Passion fruit has such a great taste, but can sometimes be a little bit tart. Agave syrup is super-sweet, so really helps balance out the flavours. Passion fruit also has a great colour… this looks like summer in a glass!

Serves 2 (drink immediately)

3 passion fruits, halved, scoop out the goodness
120ml/4fl oz/½ cup natural yogurt
2 tsp agave syrup, or to taste

1 Blend all the ingredients together with 120ml/4fl oz/½ cup ice-cold water and serve over ice.

2 Taste and add more agave syrup if it is too sharp for you.

RECEIPE
SPICY MANGO PICKLE

The best part about an Indian meal is the mango chutney.
I have always wanted to try and make it myself, but never
attempted until now. This recipe is made to eat on the same
day, otherwise the mint will go brown, so the next time you
make a curry, make this too! You need the mangos to not be
too ripe, so look out for the green ones… the sourer the
better! It isn't quite a chutney, but it's a lot fresher… and
the stuff in the supermarket probably contains quite a lot of
stuff you would rather not eat.

Makes 1 large jar (700ml/24fl oz/3 cups)

700g/1lb 9oz large green mangos
120ml/4fl oz/½ cup freshly squeezed lime juice
3 red bird's-eye chillies, slit
3 green bird's-eye chillies, slit
2 tbsp chopped mint leaves
thumb-sized piece of root ginger,
   peeled and finely grated
1 tsp cumin seeds
5 cloves
1 tsp sea salt

1 Cut each mango in half, remove the stones and discard. Leave the skins on. Take a mandolin and adjust the blade to the finest shred setting. Shred the mangos.

2 Get a 1 litre/1 quart jar. Add the lime juice, chillies, mint, ginger, cumin, cloves and salt. Seal the jar with the lid and shake to combine.

3 Add the shredded mango to the jar, seal the lid and shake several times to coat the mango completely. Allow the pickle to sit in the fridge for at least a couple of hours before serving.

SUMMER REDS

DRINK
STRAWBERRY + THYME MARGARITA

A boozy iced smoothie!

Serves 2

For the strawberry syrup
100g/3½oz/½ cup granulated
   sugar
190g/6¾oz strawberries

For the margarita
1 tbsp black lava salt,
   or sea salt
1 tbsp caster sugar
115ml/3¾fl oz/scant ½ cup lime
   juice, plus lime wedges
   to serve
115ml/3¾fl oz/scant ½ cup
   tequila
115ml/3¾fl oz/scant ½ cup
   orange liquor
leaves from 1 sprig of thyme
sliced strawberries, to serve

1 Start with the syrup. Put
   the sugar in a saucepan
   with 120ml/4fl oz/½ cup of
   water and bring to the
   boil, stirring until the
   sugar has dissolved.

Once dissolved, turn off
the heat and let it cool
completely.

2 Blend the strawberries
   with the sugar syrup
   until combined. Strain the
   mixture through a sieve,
   then pour into a blender.

3 For the margarita, mix the
   salt and sugar together and
   place on a saucer. Wipe the
   rim of 2 cocktail glasses
   with a lime wedge, then
   turn them upside down and
   dip the rims into the salt
   and sugar.

4 Pour the tequila into the
   blender with the orange
   liquor, thyme, strawberry
   syrup and lime juice, and
   tip in some ice cubes.
   Blend for 30 seconds.

5 Pour into glasses and
   garnish with sliced
   strawberries and
   lime wedges.

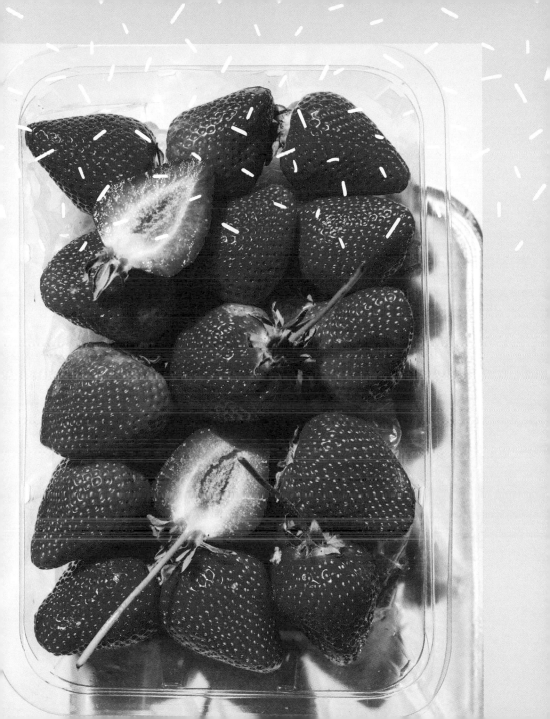

JUICE
VIRGIN MARY

Tomato juice is so very versatile and simple. You can add lots
more to it, but I think this is the perfect base for a Bloody
Mary, with the pepperiness of celery and the sweetness from
the tomatoes (be sure your mix contains cherry tomatoes).

Serves 2

750g/1lb 10 oz mixed tomatoes, including cherry tomatoes
1 celery stick

DRINK
BLOODY MARY

The world's most famous hair-of-the-dog: introducing the
Mac + Harvey Bloody Mary.

Serves 2

1 tsp Worcestershire sauce
1 x quantity Virgin Mary (see above)
1 shot of vodka, or to taste
finely grated zest of ½ unwaxed lemon
1 red chilli (seeds left in, if you want the kick),
   finely chopped
2 spears of cucumber

1 Mix the Worcestershire sauce into the Virgin Mary.
   Add 1 shot of vodka (2 if you're feeling bold).

2 Serve over ice, sprinkle lemon zest and chilli on top and
   pop a cucumber spear into each glass.

RECIPE
STRAWBERRY + VIRGIN MARY CHILLED SOUP

This is one of my favourite new recipes that I have created
for the book, using ingredients I wouldn't have usually put
together… but it works. I once had something similar when I
was on holiday, but with raspberries. This would make the best
starter for a summer's evening, or a great light lunch.

Serves 6

½ red pepper, deseeded and chopped
3 baby red sweet peppers, deseeded and chopped
1 garlic clove, crushed
½ red onion, halved and finely sliced
500g/1lb 2oz cherry tomatoes
500g/1lb 2oz strawberries, hulled,
   plus a few more to serve (optional)
250ml/9fl oz/generous 1 cup tomato juice
6 tsp balsamic vinegar

1 Chuck all the ingredients into a blender and blitz until
   almost smooth, but not completely (it's nice to have a bit
   of texture).

2 Serve in a bowl with an extra strawberry sliced on top, if
   you have any spare!

RECITE
BEAR'S SUMMER TOMATO SALAD

A simple and easy-to-make salad that is all about the quality of the ingredients. Buy the best, tastiest tomatoes you can get hold of. Using a variety of different colours and sizes of tomato will add vibrant summer colour and loads of great flavour. The same applies to the other ingredients. With the olive oil, it is worth finding one you love the flavour of, as it will add so much to the seasoning of the salad.

Serves 4 as a generous side dish

500g/1lb 2oz mixed tomatoes (a variety of colours and sizes
   gives the best flavour and looks great)
large bunch of flat-leaf parsley
2 spring onions (scallions), roughly chopped
2 large handfuls of capers, drained, rinsed
   and roughly chopped
2 large handfuls of green olives, pitted and roughly chopped
juice of 1 lemon
good-quality extra virgin olive oil
sea salt flakes and freshly ground black pepper

1 Quarter or eighth the tomatoes depending on the size, then
   run your knife through them, breaking them into smaller,
   more roughly chopped sizes. This helps to allow the flavours
   of the other ingredients marry together. Set aside in a
   colander to allow some of the water to escape from the
   tomatoes while you prepare the rest.

2 Chop the flat-leaf parsley very finely, leaving in some of the
   upper part of the stalks for added flavour and texture.

3 Combine the tomatoes, parsley, spring onions (scallions), capers and olives together and toss with your hands. Squeeze over the lemon juice, a few good glugs of the olive oil, a couple of pinches of sea salt and generous amount of black pepper and combine again. Then serve.

WATERMELONS

JUICE
WATERMELON, LIME + BASIL

Watermelon juice is a bit of a fantasy drink; they are super red in the summer months, and they make so much juice. I like to keep it simple: just add a squeeze of lime juice and serve with basil leaves. You could also add a shot of vodka!

Serves 2

½ watermelon, peeled and chopped (don't worry about the pips!)
¼ lime, zest and pith removed
2 basil leaves

1 Juice the watermelon and lime, serve with ice and a basil leaf.

JUICE
WATERMELON, STRAWBERRY, APPLE, LEMON + MINT

Watermelon juice on its own is the best, but strawberries are packed with antioxidants and are so sweet and delicious. Here, they meld with sharpness from the apple and lemon for a perfect, refreshing summery drink.

Serves 6

½ watermelon
handful of strawberries
4 Granny Smith apples, for sharpness!
½ lemon, zest and pith removed
handful of mint leaves

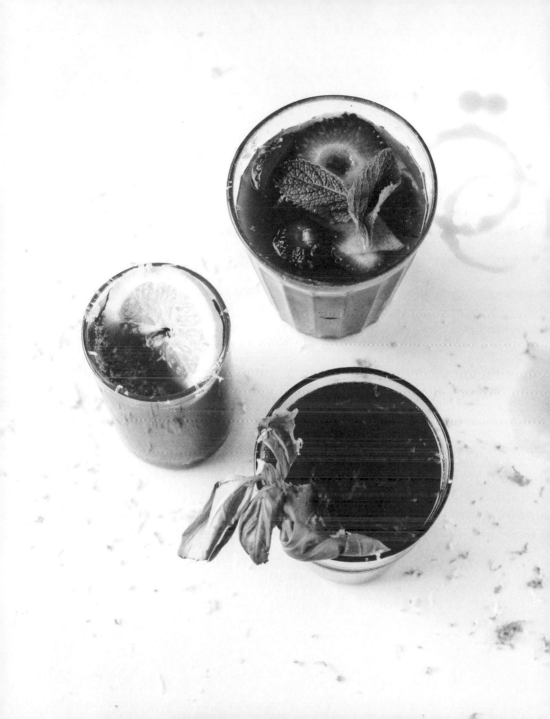

DRINK
WATERMELONADE

When watermelons come into season I can't get enough of them.
This juicy sweet-and-sour soda is a great thirst-quencher on
a hot summer's day.

Serves 8

100g/3½oz/½ cup caster (superfine) sugar
120ml/4fl oz/½ cup lemon juice
½ watermelon, juiced

1 Put the sugar in a small saucepan, pour in 120ml/4fl oz/
  ½ cup of water and bring to the boil, stirring until the
  sugar has dissolved. Set aside.

2 Mix the sugar syrup with 720ml/25fl oz/generous 3 cups of
  cold water and the lemon juice, and stir well.

3 Fill glasses with ice cubes. For each person, add 4 tbsp
  watermelon juice, then top up with lemonade. Stir gently
  before serving.

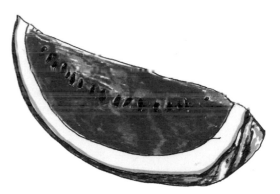

RECIPE
BEAR'S CHILLI JAM RECIPE

Bear's famous chilli jam, made by Emily and Hugo for their
rotisserie (I worked for them at Borough Market). It would
always sell out, because customers would always ask for a
dollop more. Emily was always very precious over her chilli
jam, and rightly so… I have tried them all and this is
definitely the best! Wonderful served with chicken.

Makes 6 x 200ml/7fl oz/scant 1 cup jars

250g/9oz red (bell) peppers (weight when trimmed and deseeded,
   about 2 large peppers)
150g/5½oz red chillies
   (with seeds, about 10 long red chillies)
75g/2½oz cherry tomatoes
60g/2¼oz root ginger
35g/1¼oz garlic cloves
200g/7oz canned whole plum tomatoes
500g/1lb 2oz/2½ cups golden caster (superfine) sugar
175ml/5½fl oz/scant ¾ cup cider vinegar
juice of 1 small lemon

1 Place the red peppers, chillies, cherry tomatoes, ginger, garlic and canned tomatoes into a blender and process to an even consistency. The chilli seeds should remain whole.

2 Put this all in a heavy-based saucepan, adding the sugar, vinegar and lemon juice. Stir well.

3 Bring to the boil gently, stirring at regular intervals. Once a rolling boil has been reached, skim off the scum that accumulates at the edge of the pan and keep at a rolling boil for about 5 minutes (still stirring at regular intervals to prevent sticking).

4 Reduce the heat and allow the jam to simmer gently for about 1½ hours. Ensure the jam reaches 110°C/225°F for setting point. Allow to cool a little and pour into sterilised jars (see page 159). I usually pop mine in the dishwasher and fill them hot from there.

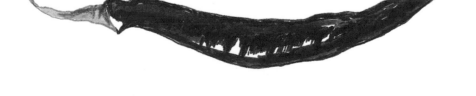

GRANITAS

A traditional granita is a semi-frozen dessert, originally from Sicily, made from sugar, water and various flavourings. I have adapted the granita to make it drinkable (and better for you), making them out of my fresh juice or blended fruit with home-made syrups. They are like slushys, but better… less slushy and more beautiful. They look like ice crystals.

DRINK
ALMOND + CHERRY GRANITA

Cherries are one of my favourite fruits. I love the combination of rich, juicy cherries with the nutty taste of almond milk.

Serves 2 (serve immediately)

100g/3½oz/½ cup granulated sugar
400ml/14fl oz/1¾ cups almond milk
200g/7oz pitted cherries

1 Place the sugar in a saucepan and pour in 120ml/4fl oz/½ cup of water. Bring to the boil, stirring until the sugar has dissolved, then remove and allow to cool.

2 Mix the sugar syrup into the almond milk and stir. Pour into a freezable, lidded container, cover and put in the freezer.

3 Freeze for 2 hours, then, with a fork, draw the ice that has formed on the edges into the centre. Put back in the freezer.

4 Repeat 3-4 times, every 30 minutes or so, until all the mixture is formed of ice crystals. Serve with the cherries.

DRINK
WATERMELON + BASIL (+ VODKA) GRANITA

Basil is such a great, summery taste and works so well with juicy watermelon. This is really refreshing and great for a hot summer's day. If you add a shot of vodka, it makes for a really tasty cocktail, too, great for a summer barbecue.

Serves 2 (serve immediately)

100g/3½oz/½ cup granulated sugar
3 sprigs of basil, plus more to serve
400ml/14fl oz/1¾ cups watermelon juice
1 shot of vodka (optional)

1 Place the sugar in a saucepan and pour in 120ml/4fl oz/½ cup of water. Bring to the boil, stirring until the sugar has dissolved. Add the basil and keep on the heat for a minute until the basil has wilted. Remove from the heat and allow to cool.

2 When completely cool, strain into a jar to remove the basil. Add the watermelon juice and stir. Pour the mix into a freezable, lidded container, cover and put in the freezer.

3 Freeze for 2 hours, then, with a fork, draw the ice that has formed on the edges into the centre. Put back in the freezer.

4 Repeat 3-4 times, every 30 minutes or so, until all the mixture is formed of ice crystals. Serve with fresh basil and a shot of vodka poured over the top.

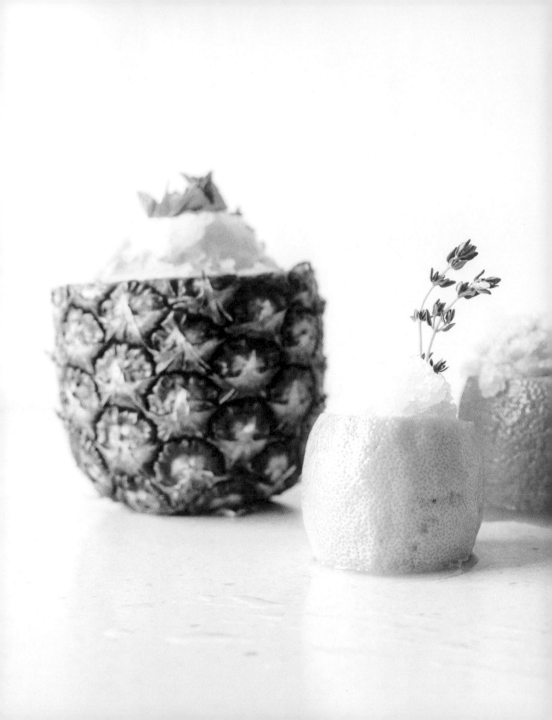

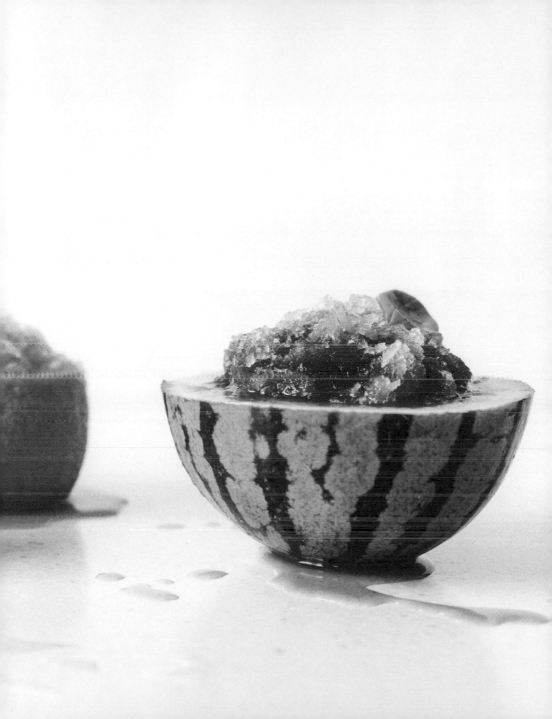

DRINK
ORANGE + CAMPARI GRANITA

Last summer's most fashionable drink seemed to be an Aperol spritz. I think this has a similar taste, but with a bit more of a tang.

Serves 2 (serve immediately)

400ml/14fl oz/1¾ cups orange juice (about 5 oranges)
1 shot of Campari

1 Juice the oranges and pour them through a sieve, to remove the 'bits'. Pour the mix into a freezable, lidded container, cover and put in the freezer.

2 Freeze for 2 hours, then, with a fork, draw the ice that has formed on the edges into the centre. Put back in the freezer.

3 Repeat 3-4 times, every 30 minutes or so, until all the mixture is formed of ice crystals. Serve with the shot of Campari poured over.

DRINK
LEMON + THYME GRANITA

Although thyme is available to buy all year round, it tends
to be much fresher and tastier in the summer. I love this
drink because the delicate flavour of the herb balances out
the zestiness of the lemon.

Serves 2 (serve immediately)

4 unwaxed lemons
100g/3½oz/½ cup granulated sugar
6 sprigs of thyme, plus more to serve

1 Zest 2 of the lemons and juice all 4.

2 Put the sugar in a saucepan and pour in 240ml/8fl oz/1 cup
  of water. Bring to the boil, stirring until the sugar has
  dissolved. Add the thyme and keep on the heat for a minute,
  then remove and allow to cool. When completely cool, strain
  to remove the herb.

3 Pour the lemon syrup into a freezable, lidded container,
  cover and put in the freezer.

4 Freeze for 2 hours, then, with a fork, draw the ice that
  has formed on the edges into the centre. Put back in
  the freezer.

5 Repeat 3-4 times, every 30 minutes or so, until all the
  mixture is formed of ice crystals.

6 Garnish with thyme to serve.

DRINK
PINEAPPLE + MINT GRANITA

Pineapple is such a summery fruit and this makes for a really refreshing drink to enjoy sitting outside with some friends. Add a shot of rum to turn this into a pineapple mojito!

Serves 2 (serve immediately)

100g/3½oz/½ cup granulated sugar
4 mint leaves, plus more to serve
400ml/14fl oz/1¾ cups pineapple juice

1 Place the sugar in a saucepan and pour in 120ml/4fl oz/½ cup of water. Bring to the boil, stirring until the sugar has dissolved. Add the mint leaves until wilted. Set aside to cool.

2 When completely cool, strain to remove the herb. Mix the pineapple juice and mint syrup in a freezable, lidded container, cover and put in the freezer.

3 Freeze for 2 hours, then, with a fork, draw the ice that has formed on the edges into the centre. Put back in the freezer.

4 Repeat 3-4 times, every 30 minutes or so, until all the mixture is formed of ice crystals. Serve with fresh mint.

DRINK
PINK GRAPEFRUIT + TARRAGON

Tarragon is something that would normally be associated with savoury food rather than sweet, but I think it goes really well with the bitterness of pink grapefruit.

Serves 2 (serve immediately)

100g/3½oz/½ cup granulated sugar
3 sprigs of tarragon
400ml/14fl oz/1¾ cups pink grapefruit juice

1 Place the sugar in a saucepan and pour in 120ml/4fl oz/ ½ cup of water. Bring to the boil, stirring until the sugar has dissolved. Add the tarragon until wilted. Set aside to cool.

2 When completely cool, strain to remove the herb. Mix the pink grapefruit juice and tarragon syrup in a freezable, lidded container, cover and put in the freezer.

3 Freeze for 2 hours, then, with a fork, draw the ice that has formed on the edges into the centre. Put back in the freezer.

4 Repeat 3-4 times, every 30 minutes or so, until all the mixture is formed of ice crystals. Serve with fresh tarragon.

ALMONDS

DRINK
ALMOND MILK

The queen of nut milks (see the Winter chapter for more
nut milk recipes - although you can make them year-round).
The taste and texture is simply delicious and, home-made, the
flavour is completely different to the stuff you can buy in
the shops. It will keep for 2 days.

Makes 1 litre/1 quart

500g/1lb 2 oz skin-on almonds

1 Put the almonds in a glass bowl, pour over 500ml/17fl oz/
  generous 2 cups of water, cover the bowl and keep chilled.

2 The next day, strain the almonds and rinse under cold
  running water.

3 Do this step in 2 batches: blend the almonds with
  1.7 litres/3 pints/7¾ cups of cold filtered water and
  strain through a nut milk bag/straining bag into a
  clean jug.

4 Keep in the fridge, in an airtight sterilised container
  (see page 159).

RECIPE
ALMOND MILK + CHERRY COMPOTE BIRCHER MUESLI

A nutty and filling breakfast that you prepare the night before. It's well worth removing the cherry stones yourself to make the delicious compote to go with the bircher.

Serves 2

80g/2¾oz jumbo (rolled) oats
300ml/10½fl oz/1¼ cups Almond
  milk (see opposite)
seeds from 1 vanilla pod
350g/12oz pitted cherries
1 tbsp honey
1 nutmeg, freshly grated
finely grated zest of
  1 unwaxed lemon

1 Soak the oats overnight in the almond milk and vanilla seeds.

2 Put the cherries in a saucepan and pour in 120ml/4fl oz/½ cup of water. Add the honey. Bring to the boil until the water evaporates and the cherries have softened. Add the nutmeg and lemon zest.

3 Serve the compote on top of the bircher.

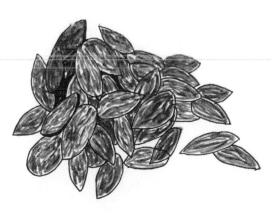

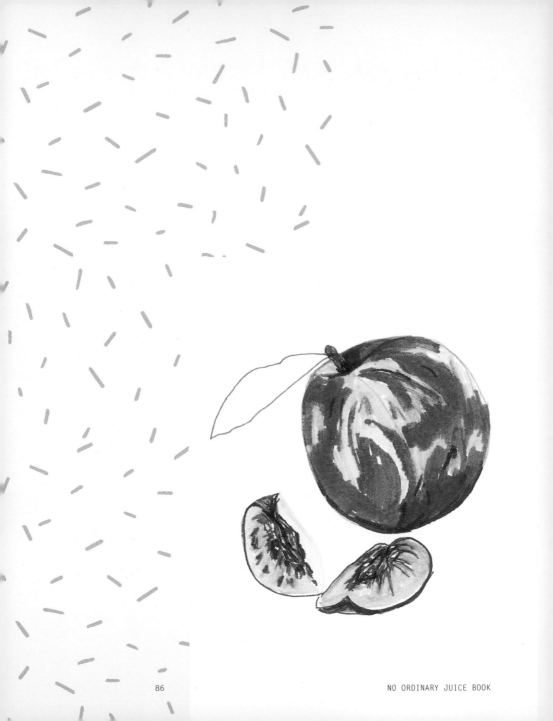

NO ORDINARY JUICE BOOK

PEACHES AND APRICOTS

JUICE
PEACH + RASPBERRY

Inspired by one of my Mum's favourite puddings, peach melba.
You could also top this up with some fizz to make the perfect
peach Bellini.

Serves 1

3 peaches, halved and pitted
60g/2¼oz raspberries
seeds from 1 vanilla pod
3 tbsp Champagne (optional)

1 Juice the peaches with the raspberries.

2 Add the vanilla seeds and Champagne (if using), and stir.

DRINK
APRICOT, ALMOND + GIN COCKTAIL

I love apricots. They are not the most practical fruits to
juice, but when they come around in summer we may as well
appreciate their wonderful fragrance while we can. This
cocktail is sweet and tangy.

Serves 2

2 apricots, pitted and quartered
1 tsp light brown sugar
115ml/3¾fl oz/scant ½ cup gin
½ tsp almond extract
juice of ¼ lime

1 In a cocktail shaker, mix the apricots and brown sugar
  until all the juices have been released. Fill the shaker
  three-quarters full with ice.

2 Add the gin and almond extract.

3 Squeeze the juice from the lime, add that and shake HARD!

4 Strain into glasses.

RECIPE
CHILLED APRICOT SOUP

A simple soup that is slightly sweet but tart. This makes a lovely starter.

Serves 4

4 apricots, pitted and
  quartered
4 tbsp agave syrup
1 tbsp finely grated unwaxed
  lemon zest

1 Put the apricots and agave syrup in a saucepan and pour in 720ml/25fl oz/ generous 3 cups of water. Place over a medium heat and bring to the boil, then reduce the heat and simmer for 15 minutes until the apricots are very soft.

2 Add most of the lemon zest and stir.

3 Purée with a hand-held blender until smooth, then set aside to cool. Chill until very cold.

4 Serve in a small glass bowl and sprinkle some of the remaining zest on top to serve.

AUTUMN

Autumn reminds me of Netil market… by which I mean
early starts with long days standing in the cold!
Autumn is a great season for hearty stews, such
as my Butternut Squash, Kale + Cashew Butter Stew
(see page 110). Bonfire Night is a highlight of the
season, so the hot juices here and small pots of
home-made beans come in handy.

Just because it's colder, it doesn't
mean salads are off the menu; autumn
is a great time of year for chicory
and courgettes, both of which are
great as a base for a salad. It's also
when our pears are at their juiciest
and sweetest, and these make a great
addition to a number of savoury dishes.

Autumn is also the time of year for
apples. When I was a child, apple
juice was my favourite, but I could
only drink it hot. Apples are low in
fructose and high in vitamin C. Their
skins contain lots of antioxidants, so
always leave them on. Apple is a great
base for any juice!

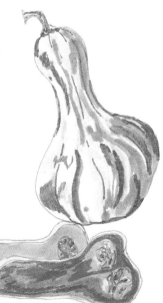

APPLES

JUICE
APPLE + CINNAMON

Everyone knows this is a winning combination. You could even
warm it up in a saucepan: apple crumble in a glass.

Serves 2

4 Cox's apples
2 tsp ground cinnamon

JUICE
APPLE, FENNEL + LIME

The sharpness of the apple and lime juice here is balanced out
by the aniseed taste of the fennel.

Serves 1

2 Granny Smith apples
1 fennel bulb
½ lime, zest and pith removed

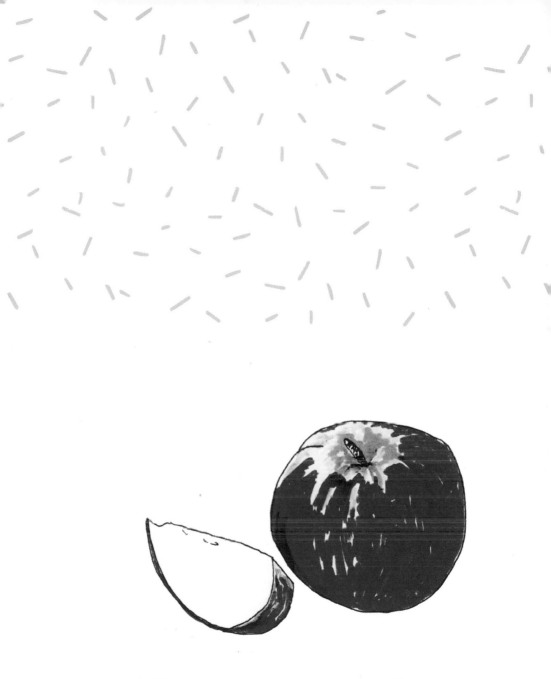

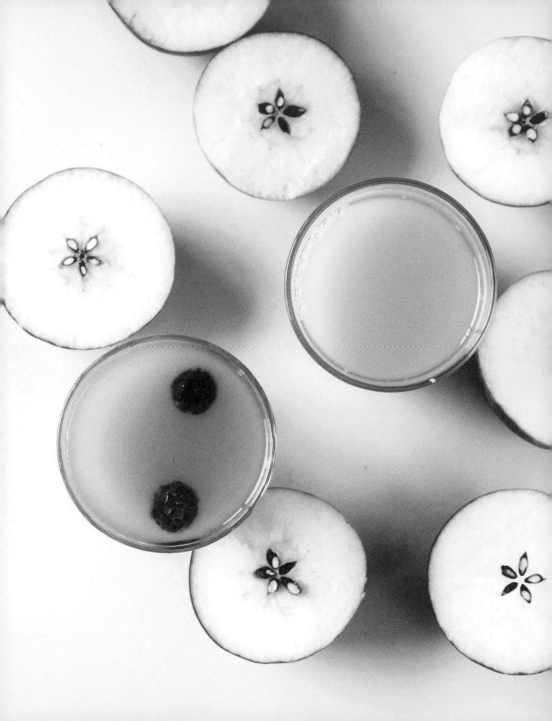

JUICE
APPLE, GINGER, LEMON +
TURMERIC

Enjoy the spiciness and knock
it back!

Serves 1

2 apples
thumb-sized piece of
    root ginger
thumb-sized piece of turmeric
½ lemon, zest and
    pith removed

JUICE
GRANNY SMITH, CUCUMBER,
CELERY, KALE, PARSLEY, LEMON
+ GINGER

If you need to hydrate and
get on a health kick, this
will do the job! Celery is a
great source of fibre and kale
is one of the best sources of
vitamin K.

Serves 1

1 Granny Smith apple
½ cucumber, skin on
1 celery stick
handful of kale,
    coarse stalks removed
handful of parsley
thumb-sized piece of
    root ginger
½ lemon, zest and
    pith removed

JUICE
APPLE, BEETROOT, GRAPEFRUIT, LEMON + GINGER

Beetroot is always quite messy, but it is worth it sometimes.
They are high in potassium and make everything purple!

Serves 4

2 apples
2 raw beetroots (beets)
1 yellow grapefruit
½ lemon, zest and pith removed
thumb-sized piece of root ginger

RECIPE
BIRCHER MUESLI WITH APPLE + FIGS

This breakfast is quick, easy and filling, and you can make
most of it the night before! Double up and make enough
for most of the working week ahead.

Serves 2

80g/2¾oz/½ cup jumbo (rolled) oats
75g/2½oz/½ cup dried figs, quartered
300ml/10½fl oz/generous 1¼ cups Apple + Cinnamon juice
  (see page 92)
1 Cox's apple
1 tsp ground cinnamon

1 Soak the oats and the figs overnight in the juice.

2 Slice the apple into circles, then slice these into strips.
  Sprinkle over the oats and figs with the cinnamon.

RECIPE
PICKLED PINK LADIES

These go really well with pork. Great in a pulled pork sarni!

Makes a 500ml/17fl oz/generous 2 cup jar

240ml/8fl oz/1 cup white wine vinegar
120ml/4fl oz/½ cup honey
pinch of sea salt
2 Pink Lady apples
3 star anise
2 tsp ground cinnamon

1 Pour 240ml/8fl oz/1 cup of water into a saucepan
  and add the vinegar, honey and sea salt. Bring it
  to the boil, then reduce the heat and simmer for
  8 10 minutes.

2 Meanwhile, core the apples without halving the
  fruits, then slice them into circles.

3 Place the apples, star anise and cinnamon in a jar
  and, once the liquid has boiled, pour it over so
  the apples are entirely covered.

4 Once cool, put the lid on and store in the fridge.
  They should keep for 1 week.

PEARS

JUICE
WILLIAM + CONFERENCE PEAR

Sweet + delicious

Serves 2

3 Conference pears
3 William pears

DRINK
PEAR SODA

A simple pear syrup with soda water, this has a lovely kick
from ginger and sweetness from maple syrup.

Serves 1

2 large pears, thinly sliced
240ml/8fl oz/1 cup maple syrup
½ tsp finely grated root ginger
soda water, to top up

1 Pour 120ml/4fl oz/½ cup of water into a saucepan and add the
  pears, maple syrup and ginger. Cook for about 30 minutes,
  until the pears soften.

2 Remove from the heat and cool to room temperature. Strain
  the liquid and save the pears (they are delicious with
  yogurt and granola).

3 Once cool, add 2-3 tbsp of the syrup to a glass, top up with
  soda water and add ice cubes.

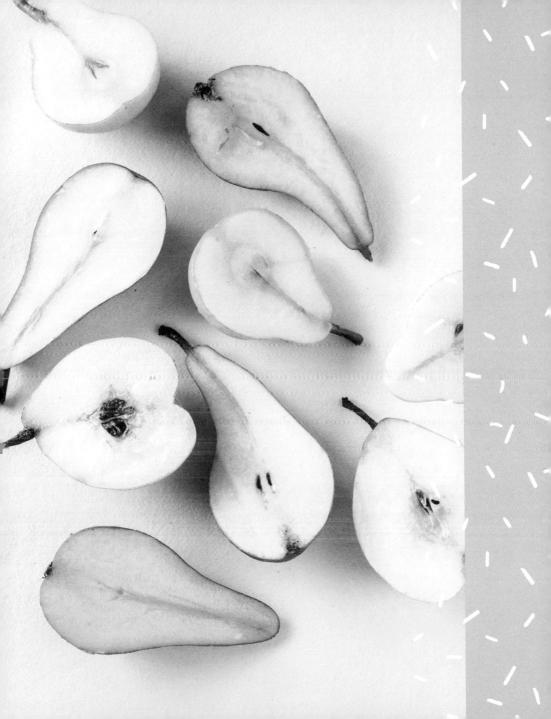

RECIPE
PEAR + CHICORY SALAD

I love chicory, but it can be a bit bitter, so I find serving
it with pears and walnuts helps to balance out the flavour.
If you can get your hands on any radicchio, mix it in with
the chicory to make the most visibly pleasing and tasty salad.

Serves 4 as a starter

100g/3½oz walnuts
3 heads of chicory, trimmed, leaves separated
2 pears, cored and quartered
3 tbsp extra virgin olive oil
1 tbsp red wine vinegar
1 tsp honey

1 Toast the walnuts in a dry frying pan over a medium heat,
  until fragrant and nicely brown; keep an eye out as the
  walnuts can burn easily. Set aside and allow to cool.

2 Place the chicory in a salad bowl, then add the pears and
  sprinkle with the toasted walnuts.

3 Mix the olive oil, vinegar and honey in a small jar and pour
  over the salad.

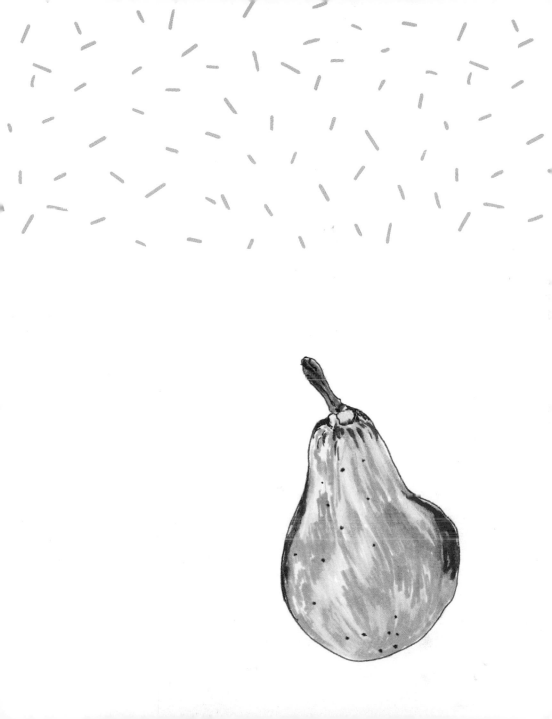

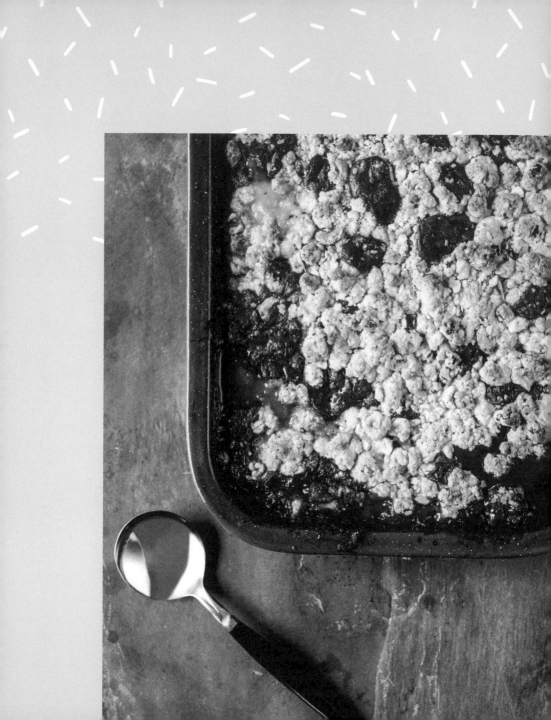

RECIPE
PEAR, GINGER, HAZELNUT + CHOCOLATE CRUMBLE

My friend Florence introduced me to this crumble. I think it's a delicious and easy pudding to share with friends.

Serves 4

For the filling
800g/1lb 12oz pears
juice of 1 lemon
thumb-sized piece of root
   ginger, finely grated
40g/1½oz/3 heaped tbsp caster
   (superfine)sugar
30g/1oz/2 tbsp unsalted
   butter

For the topping
100g/3½oz/scant 1 cup
   hazelnuts
80g/2¾oz/⅔ cup plain
   (all-purpose) flour
60g/2¼oz/⅓ cup demerara
   (turbinado) sugar
70g/2½oz/⅓ cup unsalted
   butter
60g/2¼oz chocolate (70% cocoa
   solids), chopped

1 Preheat the oven to 180°C/350°F/gas 4.

2 Peel, core and quarter the pears and place in a saucepan with the lemon juice and ginger. Cook over a medium heat until slightly softened. Mix in the caster sugar and butter, then put the pears in an ovenproof dish.

3 Now for the topping. Grind the hazelnuts in a food processor until roughly chopped, then add the flour, demerara sugar and butter. Pulse until the mix becomes a breadcrumb texture. Add 3 tsp of water and mix to create larger crumbs, then mix with the chocolate.

4 Spoon the crumble evenly over the pears and bake for 30 minutes until golden brown and bubbling.

BLUEBERRIES

JUICE
BLUEBERRY, APPLE, BASIL + LIME

Add the basil leaves last to the juice (don't put the herb
through the juicer) and let it infuse in an airtight jar or
bottle for an hour or so before drinking.

Serves 2

100g/3½oz/⅔ cup blueberries
2 apples
1 lime
2 basil leaves

RECIPE
PICKLED BLUEBERRIES + ROSEMARY

These are perfect chucked into salads, or served with cheese.

Makes a 500ml/17fl oz/generous 2 cup jar

240ml/8fl oz/1 cup white wine vinegar
50g/1¾oz/¼ cup granulated sugar
1¾ tbsp sea salt
1 tsp black peppercorns
4 sprigs of rosemary
400g/14oz/2¾ cups blueberries

1 Put the vinegar, sugar, salt, and peppercorns into a small
   saucepan and bring to the boil, stirring until the sugar
   has dissolved. Add the rosemary and simmer for a few
   more minutes.

2 Meanwhile, wash the blueberries and place into a sterilised jar (see page 159). Remove the saucepan from the heat and allow to cool slightly for about 5 minutes.

3 Pour the brine over the blueberries so they are covered. Once everything is cool, put the lid on the jar and keep in the fridge for up to 1 week.

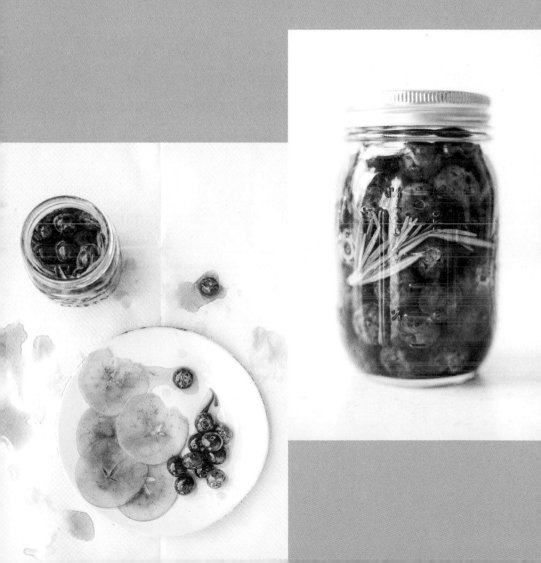

EXOTIC FRUITS

DRINK
CUSTARD APPLE LASSI

A creamy, sweet treat. You can find custard apples in most
international supermarkets.

Serves 2

1 custard apple, skinned, pips removed
120ml/4fl oz/½ cup natural yogurt
1 tsp ground cinnamon

1 Place all the ingredients in a blender with 120ml/4fl oz/
  ½ cup of ice-cold water.

2 Blend until smooth, then serve over ice.

DRINK
BANANA, LYCHEE + CARDAMOM LASSI

Lychees are one of my favourite fruits and I don't think we see enough recipes containing them. They are pretty easy to find (in most big supermarkets or international supermarkets) and balance out the heaviness and creaminess of the banana and yogurt here.

Serves 2

4 cardamom pods
1 banana, peeled and chopped
4 lychees, peeled and pitted
120ml/4fl oz/½ cup natural yogurt
½ lime, zest and pith removed
1 tsp honey

1 Bash the cardamom pods in a mortar and pestle to remove the outer husks (discard them), then grind the seeds to a powder.

2 Place all the ingredients into a blender with 120ml/4fl oz/ ½ cup of ice-cold water.

3 Blend until smooth, then serve over ice.

HARVEST FESTIVAL

JUICE
BUTTERNUT SQUASH, COURGETTE, KALE, CELERY, LEMON,
LIME + TURMERIC

This is one of my healthiest juices, great for a bit of a
detox if you've overindulged... and it tastes surprisingly good.

Serves 2

100g/3½oz piece of butternut squash, peeled and deseeded
2 courgettes (zucchini)
70g/2½oz kale, stalks discarded
3 celery sticks
1 tsp ground turmeric
½ lemon, zest and pith removed
½ lime, zest and pith removed

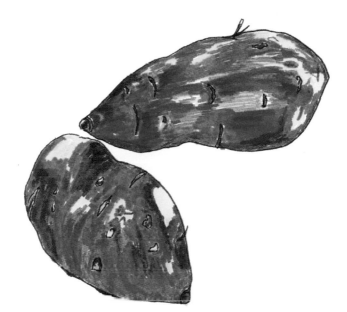

JUICE
SWEET POTATO, ORANGE, LIME + SEA SALT

Don't be put off by the sea salt in this; it actually brings
out all the sweetness in the potatoes. The sweet potato
means it's a bit more filling, but the orange and lime juice
ensure it doesn't feel too heavy.

Serves 1

1 sweet potato, peeled and chopped
1 orange, zest and pith removed
½ lime, zest and pith removed
pinch of sea salt

RECIPE
BUTTERNUT SQUASH, KALE + CASHEW BUTTER STEW

The cashew butter makes this nutty and creamy. I recommend serving it with a roti. Also I believe it is vegan.

Serves 4

2 tbsp olive oil
1 onion, finely chopped
2 garlic cloves, crushed
thumb-sized piece of root ginger, peeled and finely grated
1 butternut squash, peeled, deseeded and chopped
210g/7½oz/generous 1 cup red lentils, rinsed
4 vine tomatoes, halved
1 tsp ground cinnamon
1 tsp ground cumin
1 tsp ground turmeric
½ tsp cayenne pepper
250ml/9fl oz/generous 1 cup vegetable stock,
  plus more if needed
60g/2¼oz/¼ cup Cashew + coconut butter (see page 122)
280g/10oz kale, stalks discarded
sea salt and freshly ground black pepper
35g/1¼oz/¼ cup cashews
25g/1oz spring onions (scallions), chopped
handful of coriander (cilantro), chopped
lime wedges, to serve

1 Heat the oil in a large saucepan over a medium heat.
  Add the onion and fry until it is translucent (about
  4 minutes). Add the garlic and ginger, and continue to
  fry for a few more minutes, until the garlic is fragrant.
  Add the butternut squash, lentils, tomatoes, cinnamon,
  cumin, turmeric and cayenne pepper, and give it all a quick
  stir to combine.

2 Pour in the vegetable stock and bring to the boil. If the
  vegetables are not completely covered, add more stock so
  everything is covered by at least 2.5cm/1in of liquid.
  When everything starts to boil, reduce the heat to a simmer
  and cook for 45 minutes, or until the squash and lentils
  are very soft. Add more stock if you need it as the
  mixture cooks.

3 Add the cashew butter and stir well. Using a hand-held
  blender, blend the stew until about half of it is puréed
  and the other half still has texture. It should appear
  creamy, but chunks of the squash should still be visible.

4 Stir in the kale and let it wilt. Season to taste.

5 Serve topped with cashews, spring onions, coriander
  and lime wedges.

JUICE
HOT MULLED BEETROOT + APPLE

This is a warm, spicy and delicious drink with a deep red colour from the beetroot (beets). Perfect for Bonfire Night!

Serves 4

3 cloves
3 star anise
6 cardamom pods, crushed
1 cinnamon stick
10 juniper berries
4 black peppercorns
375ml/13fl oz/generous 1½ cups apple juice
375ml/13fl oz/generous 1½ cups beetroot (beet) juice
finely grated zest of 1 orange, plus more to serve

1 Throw all the ingredients into a saucepan placed over a medium-low heat. Don't let it boil, just heat until it is warm.

2 Take off the heat and pass through a sieve to remove all the bits.

3 Pour into nice mugs and serve with a sprinkle of orange zest on top.

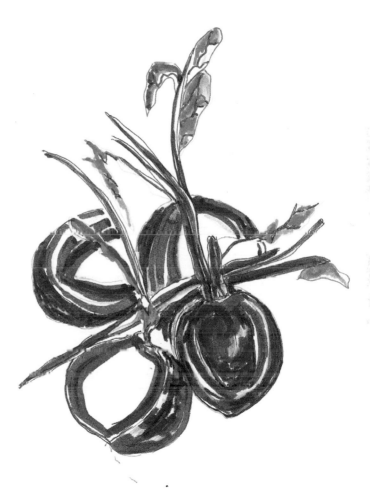

GRAPEFRUIT

JUICE
YELLOW GRAPEFRUIT +
PURPLE GRAPE

Sharp but sweet at the
same time; this is a real
favourite of mine.

Serves 2

2 yellow grapefruit,
  zest and pith removed
400g/14oz purple grapes

1 Pass through a sieve to
  remove the 'bits'.

2 Serve over ice.

JUICE
PINK GRAPEFRUIT, TANGERINE +
TURMERIC

This is a great one if you're
suffering with a cold, as
it's full of vitamin C.
Turmeric adds a really warm,
spicy flavour and is very
soothing if you have an
upset stomach.

Serves 1

1 pink grapefruit, zest and
  pith removed
1 tangerine, zest and pith
  removed
1 tsp ground turmeric

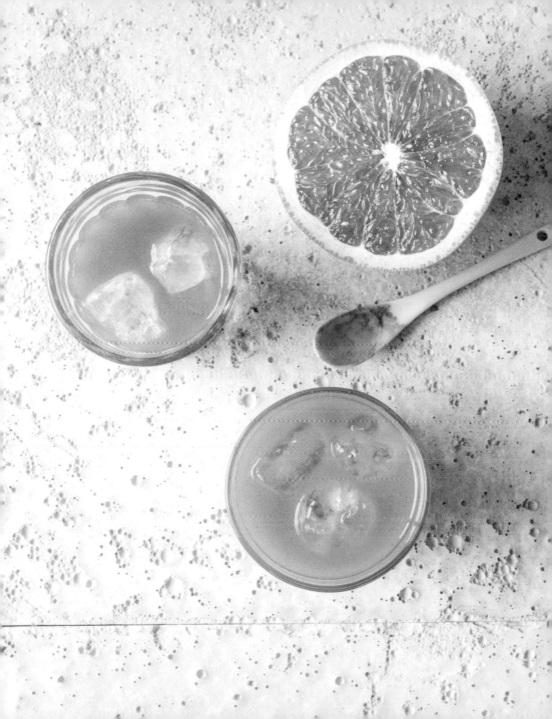

PLUMS

DRINK
PLUM + RUM COCKTAIL

This is super-easy to make, great for when you have
friends over!

Serves 1

2 ripe plum slices
60ml/2fl oz/4 tbsp dark rum
ginger beer, to top up
lime wedge

1 Mix the plum and rum together into a glass, fill with ice
   cubes and top up with ginger beer.

2 Just before drinking, squeeze in a wedge of lime.

JUICE
RAINBOW CHARD + YELLOW PLUM

Serves 2

If you can't get your hands on rainbow chard, never fear;
regular chard is just fine. The chard is quite bitter so,
with the sweet plums, it is the perfect match… with a health
kick at the same time.

6 plums, pitted
100g/3½oz rainbow chard

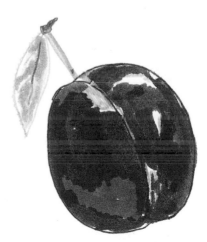

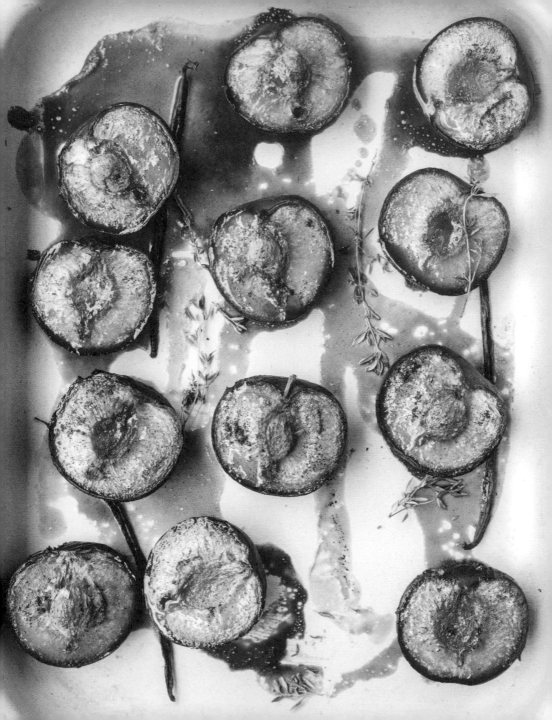

RECIPE
ROASTED PLUMS WITH THYME + VANILLA

Like all roasted fruits, this is so easy to make; a
perfect, elegant dessert for any occasion! Best served
with ice cream or yogurt.

Serves 4

6 plums, halved and pitted
1 tbsp honey
1 vanilla pod
3 sprigs of thyme
25g/1oz/2 tbsp unsalted butter

1 Preheat the oven to 180°C/350°F/gas 4.

2 Place the plums on a baking tray, cut sides up. Drizzle
  with the honey, then slit open the vanilla pod and drop
  it into the tray with the thyme. Dot the butter on top.

3 Roast for 30 minutes until soft and caramelised,
  turning halfway through. Serve with Greek yogurt.

FIGS

DRINK
FIG LASSI

Fresh ripe figs are so sweet teamed up with cinnamon in this
creamy lassi.

Serves 2

350ml/12fl oz/1½ cups natural yogurt
1 tbsp hemp seeds
4 figs
2 tbsp agave syrup
1 tsp ground cinnamon

1 Combine everything together in a blender.

2 Blend until smooth, then serve over ice.

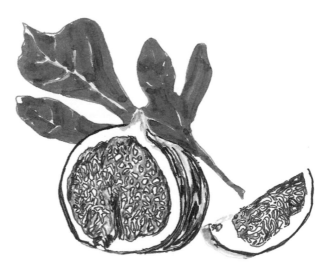

DRINK
FIG COCKTAIL

The fig season - as seems to be the case with all the most amazing fruits - is short. Using a fig jam to make this cocktail makes it extra special.

Serves 1

60ml/2fl oz/4 tbsp bourbon
1 tbsp sugar syrup (see box)
1 tbsp fig jam
juice of ½ lemon, plus more for the glass rim
demerara (turbinado) sugar, for the glass rim

1 Add the bourbon to a cocktail shaker filled with ice cubes, along with the sugar syrup, jam and lemon juice.

2 Shake until cold. Rub the rim of the cocktail glass with a lemon, then dip into a saucer of demerara sugar.

3 Strain the cocktail into the glass and serve.

TIP
To make a simple sugar syrup

Put 2 parts water and 1 part sugar in a saucepan and let it boil until the sugar has dissolved, usually around 5 minutes. Allow to cool.

AUTUMN BREAKFASTS

RECIPE
CASHEW + COCONUT BUTTER

This is a butter I made to go in one of my stews, but it actually tastes really good on toast with a bit of chopped banana, or it is a great addition to porridge.

Makes 225g/8oz

150g/5½oz unsweetened
   coconut flakes
260g/9¼oz unsalted cashews

1 Preheat the oven to
   180°C/350°F/gas 4.

2 Line a baking tray with
   baking parchment. Spread
   the coconut and cashews in
   a thin layer on the tray
   and bake for 15-20 minutes
   until golden. Allow to cool
   to room temperature.

3 Transfer the roasted
   mixture to the bowl of
   a food processor, or a
   blender. Blend until
   creamy, so it looks like
   peanut butter; it should
   take about 10 minutes.

4 Scrape into an airtight
   jar. It will keep for
   2 weeks.

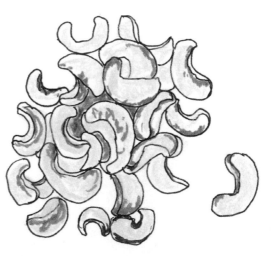

RECIPE
ADRIAN'S GRANOLA

Special K during the week and Shreddies at the weekend... my Dad was a creature of habit. Then, one day, he decided to try his hand at home-made granola and, ever since, he has been hooked. As have I. Serve with yogurt or milk of your choice and chopped fresh strawberries.

Makes 1.5kg/3lb 5oz

125g/4½oz unsalted butter
150ml/5fl oz/scant ⅔ cup
  agave syrup
1 tsp vanilla extract
500g/1lb 2oz jumbo (rolled)
  oats
100g/3½oz/scant 1 cup flaked
  almonds
100g/3½oz/scant 1 cup chopped
  hazelnuts
100g/3½oz/scant 1 cup coconut
  chips
200g/7oz/1½ cups pumpkin and
  sunflower seeds
300g/10½oz your favourite
  dried fruit

1 Preheat the oven to 140°C/ 275°F/gas 1. Have 2 large, flat baking trays to hand.

2 Melt the butter, agave syrup and vanilla gently in a saucepan. Mix all the other ingredients, except for the fruit, in a large mixing bowl. Add the melted mixture from the saucepan and stir until everything is very well combined.

3 Spread out over the baking trays. Bake for 25 minutes, turning every 5 minutes. Leave to cool completely, then mix in the dried fruit.

4 Store in a large airtight jar. It will keep for 2 weeks.

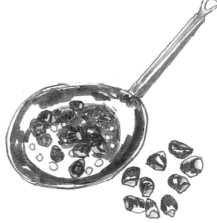

WINTER

Winter can be a long old season for all of us. Luckily,
Christmas is in the middle of it, which means a reason to
celebrate with lots of pickles, party food, winter warmers
and cocktails!

I've also included lots of juice recipes for you all to binge
on in January, to make you feel better about over-indulging…

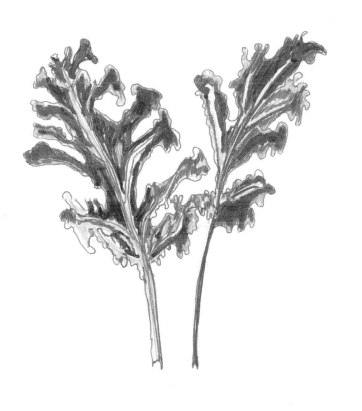

CARROTS + CLEMENTINES

JUICE
CARROT, CLEMENTINE, APPLE + GINGER

This is a classic juice combo and a Mae + Harvey bestseller.
I make it throughout the year using the sort of oranges that
are most in season at the time; this particular version uses
wintry clementines. If Christmas Eve is your favourite night,
you'll need this juice for the morning after… in fact, it's
a great pick-me-up for any morning of the party season!

Serves 4

4 medium-sized carrots
2 apples
4 clementines, zest and pith removed
thumb-sized chunk of root ginger (or more, go wild if
  you prefer)

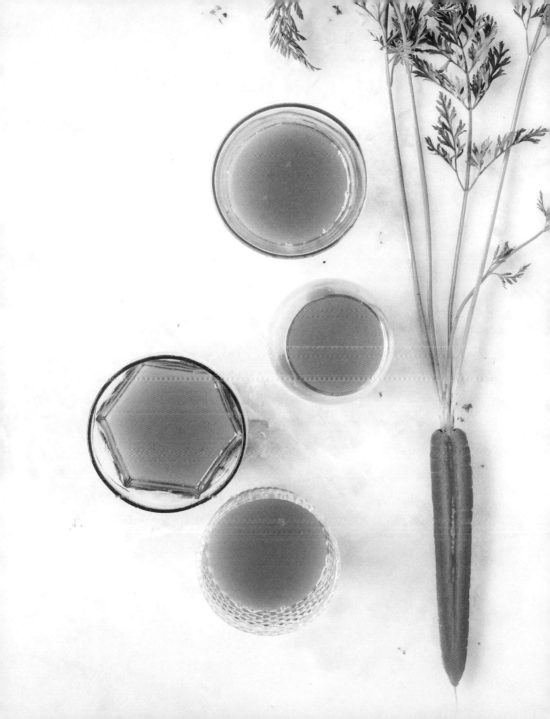

RECITE
FLORENCE'S GLUTEN-FREE CLEMENTINE, PISTACHIO + ALMOND CAKES

My friend Florence is a very talented cook and regularly chefs at Bonnington Café, a community-run place in Vauxhall that serves up vegetarian and vegan food. Florence and I mostly chat about food and I help her cook at the café; this is one of my favourite cakes that she makes. As these are baked in a muffin tray, they are the perfect size for a party!

Makes 12 muffin-sized cakes

For the cakes
4 clementines
150g/5½oz/1 cup almonds
100g/3½oz/¾ cup pistachios
6 eggs
150g/5½oz/¾ cup granulated
   sugar
1 tsp gluten-free baking
   powder
unsalted butter, for the
   muffin tray

To serve
Greek yogurt
12 clementine segments
slivered pistachios

1 Place the clementines in a saucepan, cover with water (they will float!), bring to the boil and simmer for 1 hour. Drain, leave to cool, then roughly chop the fruits, removing the seeds as you go. Preheat the oven to 180°C/350°F/gas 4.

2 Grind the nuts in a blender until fine and put into a mixing bowl. Blend the clementines to a pulp and add to the mixing bowl. Put the eggs and sugar in a food processer and mix until combined and fluffy (30 seconds to 1 minute), then add to the mixing bowl. Stir the baking powder into the mix.

3 Butter a 12-hole muffin tray and spoon the batter into the tray, leaving a 1cm gap at the top of each mould. Bake for 20 minutes, or until golden; a skewer inserted into the middle of a cake should come out clean. Turn out and leave to cool on a wire rack.

4 Once cool, serve with a blob of yogurt, a clementine segment and pistachios.

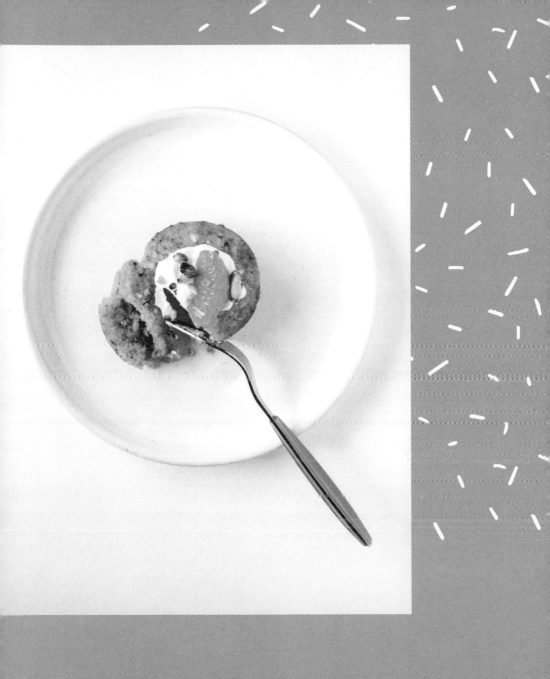

NUT MILKS

DRINK
CASHEW MILK

This is a great dairy-free alternative to milk. You can make it as smooth or textured as you like, and you can use it in lots of different ways. I came up with this particular recipe with my friend and boss Dom when we were planning the drinks menu for Lundenwic, which is where my wholesale juices are produced. We were both a bit obsessed with it for a little while! Like all nut milks, you need a bit more equipment if you want to make it at home, such as a nut milk bag/straining bag, but, as with most things, this can all be sourced online.

Because of the size of both nut milk bags and blenders, you will need to blend this recipe in batches. I also recommend that you sieve the milk again once strained, for an extra-smooth result. This will keep for two days, and you will find it separates naturally, so give it a good shake before use.

Serves 4

500g/1lb 2oz/3½ cups cashews
300g/10½oz/2½ cups pitted dates
seeds from 1 vanilla pod
pinch of sea salt
freshly grated nutmeg

1 In separate glass bowls, soak the cashews in 1 litre/
  1 quart of filtered water, and the dates in 400ml/14fl oz/
  1¾ cups of filtered water. The contents of each bowl should
  be completely covered. Leave to chill for a couple
  of hours.

2 Drain and rinse the cashews and dates, but be sure to keep
  them in separate bowls. Pour the cashews into a blender
  and cover with 600ml/21fl oz/generous 2½ cups more filtered
  water. Blend until combined, then strain the mixture
  through a nut milk bag into a large bowl or jug.

3 Blend the dates with 300ml/10½fl oz/generous 1¼ cups more
  filtered water. Strain the date mixture through the bag into
  the same bowl or jug as the cashew milk. Add the vanilla
  seeds and sea salt, then stir.

4 Transfer to a sterilised container (see page 159) to store
  in the fridge for up to 2 days. To serve, pour the mixture
  into a cup and grate the nutmeg on top.

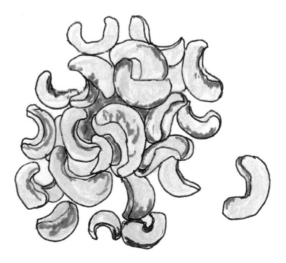

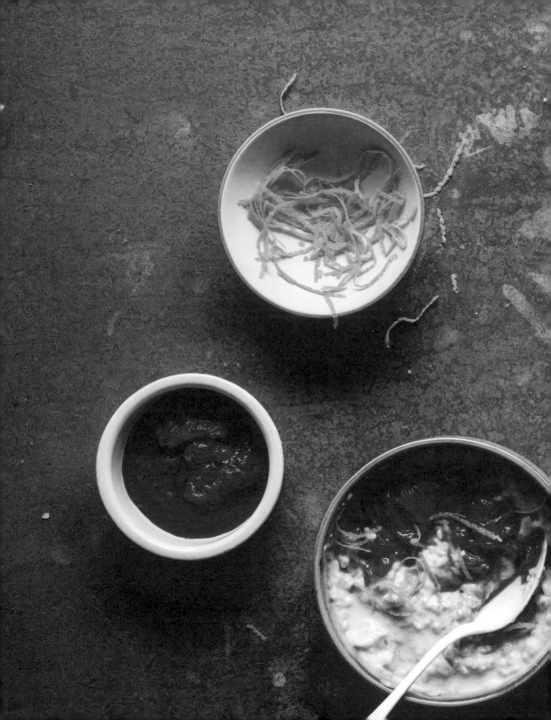

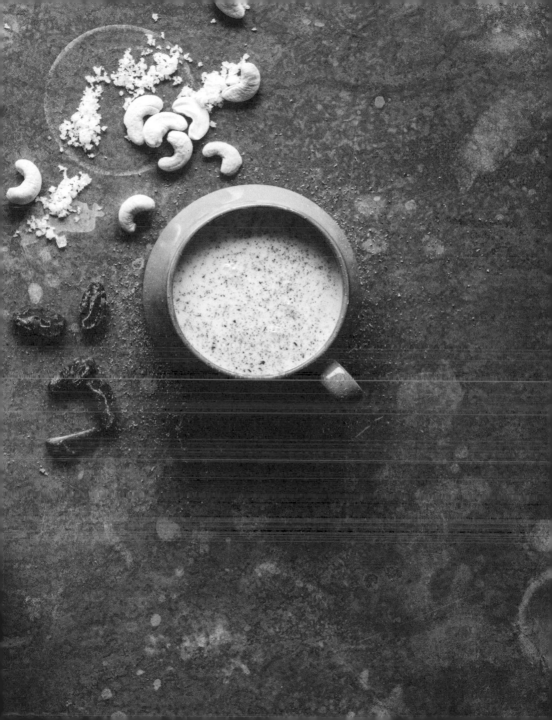

RECIPE
CASHEW MILK PORRIDGE

Cashew milk makes brilliant, extra-creamy porridge and is a really tasty variation on the traditional recipes. The secret is to cook it low and slow so you don't burn the ingredients in the pan. A bowl of this is guaranteed to make you feel happy and full in the morning.

Serves 1

40g/1½oz/¼ cup jumbo (rolled) oats
300ml/10½fl oz/generous 1¼ cups Cashew milk (see page 130)
sea salt

1 Heat up a saucepan so it's nice and warm.

2 Add the oats and cashew milk with a sprinkling of salt, then reduce the heat right down.

3 Let it cook gently for 10 minutes, until the oats are good and soft. Add more salt if you wish, then add 100ml/3½fl oz/ scant ½ cup of filtered water and continue to cook until the water has reduced and the porridge has the perfect consistency for you.

4 Serve the porridge straight away, mixing in some of my Mum's Rhubarb compote (see opposite) and sprinkling with finely grated orange zest.

RECIPE
SALLY'S RHUBARB COMPOTE

OK, so I've sort of shoe-horned this recipe in, but my Mum makes the most amazing rhubarb compote; this is one of my favourite family recipes and we always seem to have a bowl of it in the fridge. It's really versatile and can be used as the perfect topping for Cashew milk porridge (see opposite), making it very refreshing and much less heavy. It should last in the fridge for up to a week.

Serves 5

4 sticks of forced rhubarb
   (in season late February)
juice and finely grated zest
   of 1 orange
chunk of root ginger
2 tbsp brown sugar

1 Chop the rhubarb into chunks and place in a saucepan over a low heat. Add the orange juice and zest, then grate the ginger into the pan. Add 3-4 tbsp of water and the sugar.

2 Heat for 5-10 minutes, but don't let it boil!

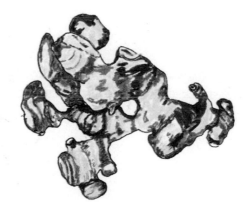

DRINK
HOT ALMOND MILK WITH ROSEMARY, CRANBERRY + VODKA

I think this recipe sums up what this book is about: creating
delicious drinks, enjoying them, then combining any extra
bits with other ingredients to make an entirely new taste
experience. I tasted something similar to this in Gothenburg
at a Christmas market and loved it, so I wanted to recreate it
for you all to try.

Serves 4

500ml/17fl oz/generous 2 cups Almond milk (see page 130)
3 tbsp Cranberry jelly (see page 138)
100ml/3½fl oz/7 tbsp port
3 tsp honey
2 sprigs of rosemary
200ml/7fl oz/scant 1 cup vodka

1 Over a low heat, simmer the almond milk, cranberry jelly,
   port, honey and 1 sprig of rosemary, stirring occasionally
   until the cranberry jelly has fully melted.

2 Add about 3 tbsp of the vodka to each of 4 mugs and divide
   the warm almond milk mixture on top. This next bit is
   optional: cut the remaining sprig of rosemary into 4, light
   each piece, then set it on fire before you add it to the
   mugs to serve.

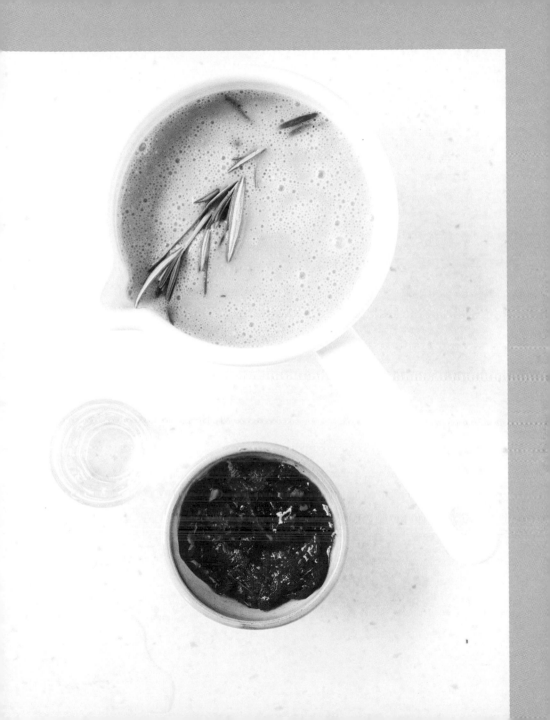

RECIPE
CRANBERRY JELLY

Christmas time doesn't make sense without cranberry jelly: an essential. Add this to your cocktail mixes and your turkey!!

Makes 1 jar

275g/9¾oz cranberries
¼ tsp ground cinnamon
⅛ tsp ground nutmeg
pinch of ground cloves
300g/10½oz/1½ cups granulated sugar
160ml/5¼fl oz/⅔ cup apple cider
juice of ½ lemon

1 Place the cranberries in a medium saucepan. Mix the spices into the sugar, then add the sugar mixture to the cranberries and stir to combine.

2 Pour in the cider and lemon juice.

3 Cook over a medium-high heat, stirring regularly. Once the cranberries have burst and the sauce has thickened, remove the pan from the heat. (If the sauce seems too thick, just add a splash of water.)

4 Push the mix through a fine sieve into a bowl, until all that's left in the sieve are bits of seeds and skins. Pour the strained sauce into a sterilised jar (see page 159).

5 Place the lid on top and let the jelly set in the fridge for at least 12 hours before consuming.

DRINK
BRAZIL + HAZELNUT MILK

Once you know the basic method of making nut milk, you
can create loads of different types. This milk is a great
complement to any smoothie; I like to add banana and cacao
powder to make a chocolate banana milkshake.

Makes 250ml/9fl oz/generous 1 cup

150g/5½oz/1 cup brazil nuts
150g/5½oz/1¼ cups hazelnuts
sea salt

1 Soak the nuts overnight in 100ml/3½fl oz/7 tbsp of filtered
  water and a pinch of salt.

2 Drain the nuts and rinse them, throwing away the
  soaking water.

3 Place the nuts into a blender and pour in 1 litre/1 quart
  of fresh filtered water. Blend for about 1 minute until
  white and creamy.

4 Place a nut milk bag inside a large bowl, hold on to both
  sides and carefully pour the nut mixture into it. You may
  want to do this in 2 stages, depending on the size of your
  nut milk bag.

5 The mix will start to come out of the bottom and look
  beautiful. Squeeze the bag until all that remains of the
  ground nuts within it is a dry pulp.

BLOOD ORANGES

JUICE
HOT BLOOD ORANGE

When Mae + Harvey first got started, I had a stall at Netil
Market in London Fields. In winter, when it was freezing cold,
I made hot juices to sell at the stall. The simplicity of this
blood orange juice spiced up with cinnamon and star anise was
- and still is - the perfect winter warmer. It's also a great
alternative to mulled wine.

Serves 8

juice of 10 blood oranges
2 cinnamon sticks
3 star anise
freshly grated cinnamon, to serve (optional)

1 Pour the blood orange juice into a saucepan, then add the
  cinnamon and star anise.

2 Gently warm the juice, taking it off the heat before
  it boils.

3 Get cosy with your friends and enjoy a big mug of the
  hot juice together, sprinkling the mugs with cinnamon,
  if you like.

JUICE
BLOOD ORANGE, TANGERINE, POMEGRANATE, PEAR + GINGER

This is delicious and best enjoyed first thing in the morning. With the pomegranate, tap all the seeds out into a bowl first (see page 146), then save the juice that surrounds them to add to the drink. You can then store the seeds in the fridge, or have them sprinkled on top of your yogurt in the morning.

Serves 4

2 blood oranges, zest and pith removed
3 tangerines, zest and pith removed
2 pears
thumb-sized piece of root ginger
juice from ½ pomegranate

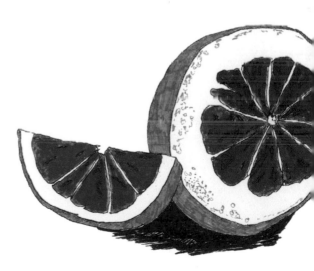

DRINK
BLOOD ORANGE MIMOSAS

Very elegant, so simple yet delicious. Go heavy with the
chilled Prosecco… but not too heavy, or you'll lose the
delicate tang of the juice. The blood oranges give this drink
a wonderful red glow, and a final sprinkling of zest adds to
the overall bitter balance.

Serves 1

50ml/1½fl oz/generous 3 tbsp chilled blood orange juice
Prosecco
finely grated zest of 1 blood orange

1 Pour the blood orange juice into a cocktail glass and top
  up with chilled Prosecco.

2 Add a twist of blood orange zest, grate a little sprinkling
  more on top and serve.

3 Multiply the recipe by 20 and have a mimosa party!

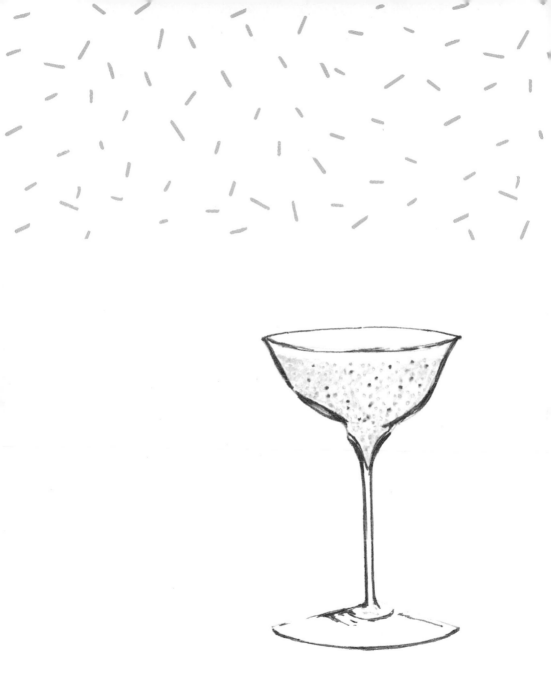

RECIPE
AUNTY MAXINE'S MARMALADE

'Aunty Maxine makes marvellous marmalade.' Grandma

My great Aunty Maxine makes marmalade, and she wrote me a
letter from Leeds with the recipe on. She told me that you
have to be quick when it comes to buying Seville oranges
as they aren't around for very long (from about the end of
December to mid-February). You can only make marmalade with
Seville oranges because they are bitter (not great for juicing
though!). Place a glass in the fridge before you start.

This amount will make 1.8-2.25kg/4-5lb

900g/2lb Seville oranges
2 lemons
900g/2lb granulated sugar

1 Wash all the fruit and place it all in a very large
   saucepan, preferably a preserving pan.

2 Add 2.25 litres/4 pints of water, bring to the boil, cover
   and cook for about 1 hour, or until the oranges are soft
   enough to be puréed. Strain the fruit over a large bowl,
   reserving the liquid.

3 Cut the fruit in half and scoop out the pulp and seeds.
   Put these into a pan with another 600ml/21fl oz/
   generous 2½ cups of fresh water, bring to the boil and
   simmer for 10 minutes. Strain over the bowl containing
   the liquid from the first boiling.

4 Cut the fruit zests into thin strips and put them into a
   measuring jug. Add all the liquid and then make the amount
   up to 2.25 litres/4 pints again with water. (Some will have
   boiled off during cooking.)

5 Return the mixture to a preserving pan or large saucepan, bring to the boil, add the sugar, then return to the boil and boil until a set is reached (see below); about 1 hour.

6 Pot immediately into sterilised jars (see page 159) and cover. The marmalade will only last for about a week because it is delicious on porridge and - of course - on toast. However, if you're not as greedy as my family, Maxine has told me it will last up to 6 months in the fridge.

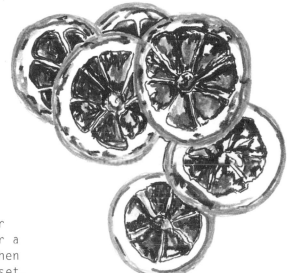

TO TEST FOR A SET

While you're making your preserve, put a glass or a saucer in the fridge. When you want to test for a set, fetch the glass or saucer from the fridge and put in a spoonful of the marmalade or jam. Return it to the fridge and, after 5 minutes, the surface should wrinkle if gently pushed.

POMEGRANATES

DRINK
HOME-MADE GRENADINE

A little fact for you: the name 'grenadine' originated from the French word *grenade* which means pomegranate! Grenadine is non-alcoholic syrup made from pomegranate juice, which is tart but is sweetened by sugar to add flavour and colour to cocktails.

Makes about 300ml/10½fl oz/ generous 1¼ cups

240ml/8fl oz/1 cup pomegranate juice, at room temperature
200g/7 oz/1 cup granulated sugar

Combine the pomegranate juice with the sugar in a jar and give it a really good shake until the sugar has dissolved. Store in the fridge; this keeps for at least 1 week.

DRINK
SHIRLEY TEMPLE BLACK

The original Shirley Temple drink was created by a bartender in Honolulu in the 1930s, at a place visited by the child actress herself. This version is alcoholic… but it's still sweet and colourful!

Serves 2

500ml/17fl oz/generous 2 cups soda water
3 tbsp Aperol
2 tbsp Home-made grenadine (see left)
1 tbsp fresh lime juice, plus lime wheels to serve
2 drops of orange bitters, or to taste

1 Combine the soda water, Aperol, grenadine and lime juice in a jug. Stir gently to mix.

2 Taste and add the orange bitters.

3 Divide between 2 glasses and serve over ice with a wheel of lime for garnish.

JUICE
HOT HIBISCUS + POMEGRANATE

Hibiscus is well known for its colour, tanginess and flavour.
The pomegranate here complements the hibiscus flowers, making
a refreshing and warming drink that will make you feel as
tropical as the hibiscus flowers for a few minutes!

Serves 4

50g/1¾oz dried hibiscus flowers
thumb-sized piece of root ginger, finely chopped
1 cinnamon stick, plus more to serve
1 litre pomegranate juice
agave syrup, to taste

1 Put the hibiscus flowers, ginger and cinnamon into a large
  saucepan with the pomegranate juice and 200ml/7fl oz/scant
  1 cup of water. Bring slowly to the boil, then reduce the
  heat and simmer for 2 minutes.

2 Turn the heat off and allow to infuse for 10 minutes.
  Strain through a sieve and pour into glasses. Serve warm
  with a cinnamon stick, offering the agave syrup for people
  to add to taste.

WINTER BERRIES

DRINK
WINTER BERRY CORDIAL

Cordial, or squash (!), was always very popular in our house, but I had never really experimented with making my own until now. You can enjoy this not only with ice and water, but also mulled (see page 150). You will have some blackberries left over, which you could use to make compote.

Makes 1.2 litres/generous 2 pints/5 cups

1kg/2lb 4oz blackberries
500g/1lb 2oz caster (superfine) sugar
2 star anise

1 Put the blackberries in a large bowl, cover with plenty of water and give them a rinse. Drain the blackberries and put them in a saucepan with 1.5 litres/9 pints of fresh cold water. Place over a medium-high heat and bring to the boil for 10 minutes.

2 Using a nut milk bag, or a clean tea towel over a colander, strain the fruit over a clean bowl or saucepan for around 45 minutes; do not squeeze the bag or the cordial will be cloudy.

3 Once strained, add the sugar and star anise to the strained blackberry juice and bring to the boil in a large saucepan, skimming off any froth that may surface. Boil for 10 minutes over a medium-high heat.

4 Remove the star anise and pour the cordial into sterilised bottles or jars (see page 159); it should last for up to 3 months.

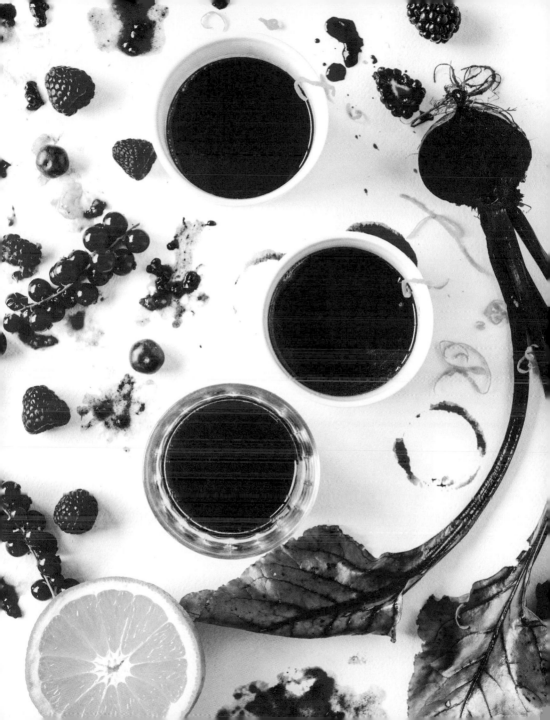

DRINK
MULLED ORANGE + BERRY CORDIAL

Mulled wine is the winter season classic. This non-alcoholic version looks like the real thing and still tastes delicious.

Serves 6

1 orange
½ lemon
1 clementine
8 cloves
175ml/5½fl oz/scant ¾ cup Winter berry cordial (see page 148)
300ml/10½fl oz/generous 1¼ cups orange juice
½ tbsp agave syrup
4 tbsp honey, or to taste
1 cinnamon stick
2 star anise
½ tsp ground ginger

1 Cut the orange into quarters and the half-lemon in half, then slice the quarters.

2 Stud the clementine with the cloves, then put all the ingredients into a large saucepan. Pour in 1 litre/1 quart of water, stir and bring to the boil, then reduce the heat and simmer for 15-20 minutes.

3 Taste and add more honey if needed.

JUICE
BEETROOT, WINTER BERRY +
ORANGE

Beetroot juice has a very
distinctive taste, and people
can find it quite difficult to
drink, which is why I like
to combine it with delicate
and sweet-tasting fruits.
You could use raspberries,
blueberries, strawberries
or blackberries here. Any
types of berry work, in
fact, so just use whatever
is available to you in your
winter. Even frozen berries
are fine, as long as you
remember to defrost them the
night before.

Serves 2

1 large orange, zest and
  pith removed
large handful of berries
3 raw beetroots

JUICE
BEETROOT, PARSNIP + APPLE

With this recipe, I was
trying to prove to stockists
that juice isn't just a
summer thing. Parsnips,
those stalwart winter
root vegetables, make a
surprisingly great juice that
is quite thick and spicy…
give it a go!

Serves 2

3 raw beetroots
1 large parsnip
1 apple

JUICE
MULLED APPLE CIDER WITH
ORANGE + PEAR

This is a mellow recipe
where the apple cider can be
replaced by apple juice, for
a non-alcoholic version.

Serves 8

1 pear
1 orange
2 tbsp cloves
1 lemon
4 allspice berries
thumb-sized piece of root
  ginger, cut into
  small pieces
1 medium cinnamon stick
2 litres apple cider

1 Stud the pear and orange
  with cloves and, using
  a vegetable peeler, peel
  large pieces of zest from
  the lemon, avoiding the
  white pith.

2 Put all the fruits and
  spices into a medium-sized
  saucepan over a low heat.
  Pour the apple cider over
  and allow to simmer for at
  least 30 minutes.

3 Serve hot, in mugs.

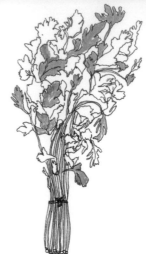

JUICE
ORANGE, APPLE, SPINACH,
PARSLEY + GINGER

I always think orange is the
best base for any juice,
especially when parsley is
involved… which is definitely
an acquired taste! Parsley
is rich in vital vitamins
and known to flush out excess
fluids from the body, which
you will probably need
around Christmas.

Serves 2

1 large orange, zest and
  pith removed
2 apples
large handful of spinach
handful of parsley
thumb-sized chunk of
  root ginger

JUICE
PERSIMMON MOJITOS

We can be tropical even in winter with this mojito!!

Serves 2

For the persimmon syrup
flesh of 2 persimmons (seeds and skins removed)
85g/3oz/scant ½ cup brown sugar
1 tsp ground cinnamon
1 tsp ground ginger
1 tsp ground nutmeg
1 tsp cloves
seeds from 1 vanilla pod

For the mojito
6 mint leaves, plus more to serve
finely grated zest and juice of 1 lime
120ml/4fl oz/½ cup persimmon syrup
2 shots of spiced rum (4 if you want double measures)
soda water

1 Start with the syrup. Put the persimmon flesh into a saucepan over a medium heat and add the brown sugar and spices (except the vanilla). Pour in 360ml/12fl oz/1½ cups of water, bring to the boil and simmer for 5 minutes. Remove from the heat and stir in the vanilla seeds. Allow to cool.

2 Once cooled, sieve the syrup into a bottle or glass jar to remove any stringy bits of flesh.

3 Now for the mojitos. In a mortar and pestle, bash the mint with the lime zest, then put them in a small jug. Stir in the lime juice, persimmon syrup and rum. Add a few ice cubes to 2 mojito glasses, pour in the rum mixture and top up with soda water. Serve with fresh mint.

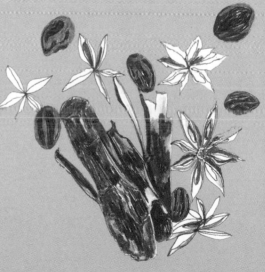

RECIPE
PERSIMMON + POMEGRANATE WINTER FRUIT SALSA

This recipe is a perfect side salad, or it even works as a dip for tortilla chips. Think of it as guacamole with an added twist!

Serves 2

juice of 2 limes
1 tsp sea salt
2 shallots, finely chopped
2 persimmons, peeled, seeds removed
1 large avocado, peeled and pitted
1 large pomegranate
1 tsp ground cinnamon
3 sage leaves, finely chopped
large handful of mint, chopped

1 Combine the lime juice, salt and shallots in a bowl. Set aside while you prepare the rest of the ingredients.

2 Finely chop the persimmon and avocado and add to the bowl.

3 Chop the pomegranate in half and – over a glass bowl filled halfway with water – pat the seeds out with a spoon, holding the pomegranate halves cut sides down. (Those that float are the good ones.) Pick out the floating seeds and add to the rest of the ingredients.

4 Add the cinnamon, sage and mint. Combine it all together and allow 30 minutes before serving, so all the flavours can develop.

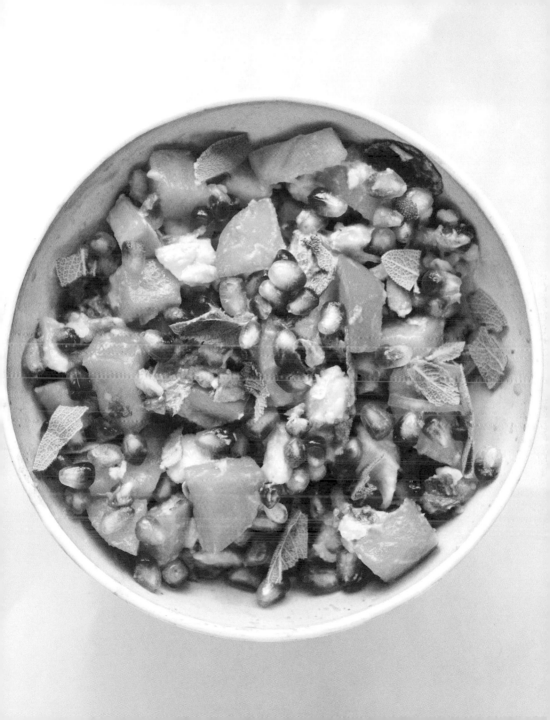

INDEX

NO ORDINARY JUICE BOOK

THANKS

I want to say thank you to everyone who has helped me to create this book. After my first meeting with Pavilion I rang my Mum immediately and told her. I couldn't believe it, and genuinely thought it was a joke. When it sunk in, I said to her, 'I'll be able to do a thank you page!' So here goes…

Firstly, thank you to Emily Preece-Morrison, Krissy Mallett and Katie Cowan at Pavilion for approaching me and the work you have put into this book; and to the photographers Liz and Max, stylist Charlie Phillips, editor Lucy Bannell, and the designers Laura Russell and Zoe Anspach. It has been a brilliant experience and I hope the readers get as much enjoyment from the book as we did making it.

My family have been and always will be a fundamental part of it all. Mum, Dad, Alex and George, thank you for taking me seriously. For helping me peel oranges, scoop melons and pick the stones out of the cherries. For loading and unloading the car, standing in the rain at the markets, storing glass bottles, telling everybody we know about the juices and being my biggest fans.

I also want to thank my Grandpa Eric; he knows what he's done and he is a very special man. And of course my lovely Grandma who makes the best orange juice in the world.

A big thank you, too, to all my friends who have helped along the way. And special thanks to artist Lis Byrd and designer Kenny Foot who have helped create Mae + Harvey.